ANESTHESIOL

PRETEST® SELF-ASSESSMENT AND REVIEW

ANESTHESIOLOGY

PRETEST® SELF-ASSESSMENT AND REVIEW

Second Edition

Edited by

Saundra E. Curry, M.D.
Associate Professor of Anesthesiology
College of Physicians and Surgeons
Columbia University
New York, New York

Contributors

Matthew Levine, M.D.
Assistant Professor of Anesthesiology

J. Stephen Mercer, M.D.
Assistant Professor of Anesthesiology

Wendy Silverstein, M.D.
Assistant Professor of Anesthesiology

Lena Sun, M.D.
Associate Professor of Anesthesiology
Associate Professor of Pediatrics

College of Physicians and Surgeons
Columbia University
New York, New York

McGraw-Hill
Health Professions Division
PreTest® Series

New York   St. Louis   San Francisco   Auckland   Bogotá   Caracas   Lisbon   London   Madrid
Mexico City   Milan   Montreal   New Delhi   San Juan   Singapore   Sydney   Tokyo   Toronto

McGraw-Hill

A Division of The McGraw·Hill Companies

Anesthesiology: PreTest® Self-Assessment and Review, 2/e

1 2 3 4 5 6 7 8 9 0 DOCDOC 9 9 8 7

ISBN 0-07-015102-4

The editors were John Dolan and Peter McCurdy.
The production supervisor was Helene G. Landers
The cover design is by Jim Sullivan, RepoCat Graphics
    and Editorial Services.
R.R. Donnelley & Sons was printer and binder.
The book was set in Times Roman by Digitype.

Library of Congress Cataloging-in-Publication Data

Anesthesiology : PreTest self-assessment and review / edited by
    Saundra E. Curry : contributors, Matthew Levine . . . [et al.].—2nd
    ed.
        p. cm.
    Includes bibliographical references.
    ISBN 0-07-015102-4
    1. Anesthesiology—Examinations, questions, etc.   I. Curry,
Saundra E.   II. Levine, Matthew.
    [DNLM: 1. Anesthesiology—examination questions. WO 218.2 A5785
1998]
RD82.3.A5   1998
617.9′6′076—dc21
DNLM/DLC
for Library of Congress   97-25675
                                                              CIP

CONTENTS

PREFACE

The first edition of this book was quite successful, as these things go. The amount of work that was required to pull it all together was so great, however, that we dreaded the inevitable phone calls telling us that another edition was due. But here it is, written again for our residents whose comments were taken to heart when we revised the questions. The most common criticism was that after studying from this book they felt compelled to read more! In the preface for the first edition we stated that this was precisely what we hoped would happen, so we don't see that as a negative criciticism at all. The questions remain challenging, and difficult, commensurate with the level of expertise expected on the anesthesia written board exam, so our residents tell us. In fact, our residents have told us

that our book is more difficult than others of its kind on the market. They say that they studied from others, felt comfortable, turned to ours and realized they still had a lot to learn. We have updated references to reflect both new book editions and new information that has come out since 1993.

Again, we would like to thank many people for their help in getting this second edition completed. Our families were tolerant of late nights and weekend work. Susan Noujaim kept on the pressure so that we were only one year behind, instead of two! And finally NiTanya Nedd collated data from five very different authors and typed, organized and computerized the entire project.

INTRODUCTION

Anesthesiology: PreTest® Self-Assessment and Review, 2/e provides residents and practitioners with a comprehensive and convenient instrument for self-assessment and review within the field of anesthesiology. The 550 questions parallel the format and degree of difficulty of the questions contained in the anesthesiology written boards.

Each question in the book is followed by an answer, a paragraph explanation, and a specific page reference to a textbook. A bibliography listing the sources used in the book follows the last chapter.

Perhaps the most effective way to use this book is to allow yourself one minute to answer each question in a given chapter; as you proceed, indicate your answer beside each question. By follow-ing this suggestion, you will be approximating the time limits imposed by the board examinations previously mentioned.

When you finish answering the questions in a chapter, you should then spend as much time as you need verifying your answers and carefully reading the explanations. Although you should pay special attention to the explanations for the questions you answered incorrectly, you should read *every* explanation. The editor and contributors of this book have designed the explanations to rein-force and supplement the information tested by the questions. If, after reading the explanations for a given chapter, you feel you need still more infor-mation about the material covered, you should consult and study the references indicated.

ANESTHESIOLOGY

PRETEST® SELF-ASSESSMENT AND REVIEW

PHARMACOLOGY

Directions: Each question below contains four or five suggested responses. Select the **one best** response to each question.

1. Opioid effects on respiratory rate and rhythm include all the following EXCEPT
   - (A) decreased respiratory rate
   - (B) irregular respiratory rate
   - (C) Cheyne-Stokes breathing patterns
   - (D) increased respiratory pauses
   - (E) delays in expiration

2. Factors that increase the magnitude of opioid-induced respiratory depression include all the following EXCEPT
   - (A) bolus injections of opioids
   - (B) increased age
   - (C) concomitant use of benzodiazepines
   - (D) decreased hepatic blood flow
   - (E) increased clearance with decreased volume of distribution

3. All the following statements concerning opioids and their effects on the endocrine system's response to stress are true EXCEPT
   - (A) the mechanism by which opioids attenuate the endocrine stress response is not totally known
   - (B) opioids may decrease the endocrine stress response by decreasing nociceptive input
   - (C) opioids may decrease the endocrine stress response via centrally mediated neuroendocrine responses
   - (D) opioids may affect nociception at several different levels of the central nervous system
   - (E) opioids increase blood level of anabolic hormones such as insulin and testosterone during stress

4. All the following statements concerning opioids and sensory evoked potentials are true EXCEPT

- (A) brainstem auditory evoked potentials are minimally affected by opioids
- (B) somatosensory evoked potentials (SSEPs) are minimally affected by opioids
- (C) meperidine is unique among the narcotics in its ability to alter latency and amplitude of SSEPs
- (D) the effect of opioids on SSEPs is dose-dependent
- (E) continuous infusion of opioids affects SSEPs minimally

5. All the following statements about opioids are true EXCEPT

- (A) neuroleptanesthetic preparation of droperidol and fentanyl citrate (Innovar) provides analgesia and maintenance of cardiovascular stability but should not be used in patients being treated for Parkinson's disease
- (B) continuous infusion of narcotic provides decreased total dose but more pain in the immediate postoperative period when compared with intermittent boluses
- (C) studies support the fact that sufentanil gives greater intraoperative hemodynamic stability compared with fentanyl
- (D) transdermal and transmucosal applications of opioids have become accepted though not always reliable modes of delivery
- (E) opioids administered prior to induction may potentiate the cardiodepressant effects of induction agents such as thiopental

6. All the following are side effects of meperidine EXCEPT that it

- (A) increases coronary artery blood flow
- (B) may act as a negative inotrope
- (C) may elicit histamine release more frequently than do other opioids
- (D) may cause an increase in heart rate because of structural similarities to atropine
- (E) may cause CNS toxic effects

7. All the following properties concerning the opioid remifentanil are true EXCEPT

- (A) remifentanil is unique because it does not cause respiratory depression
- (B) chest wall rigidity can result in a dose-dependent fashion
- (C) remifentanil has a half-life of 10 min
- (D) remifentanil is rapidly metabolized by nonspecific plasma and tissue esterases
- (E) side effects of remifentanil include pruritis and nausea and vomiting

8. All the following statements are true EXCEPT

- (A) compared with fentanyl, sufentanil has a smaller volume of distribution and a shorter elimination half-life and is more lipophilic
- (B) opioids produce respiratory depression through a direct action on brainstem respiratory centers
- (C) potential side effects of naloxone include hypertension, pulmonary edema, and cardiac arrest
- (D) alfentanil has a short duration of action because it has the highest clearance of any of the commonly used opioids

9. Potent inhaled agents may potentially cause renal dysfunction in all the following cases EXCEPT

   (A) metabolism of sevoflurane by the liver may lead to nephrotoxic levels of inorganic fluoride (F^-)

   (B) metabolism of desflurane by the liver may lead to nephrotoxic levels of F^-

   (C) metabolism of halothane by the liver may lead to nephrotoxic levels of F^-

   (D) metabolism of enflurane by the liver may lead to nephrotoxic levels of F^-

   (E) metabolism of methoxyflurane by the liver may lead to nephrotoxic levels of F^-

10. Which of the following inhaled agents has been shown to be mutagenic in humans?

   (A) Enflurane
   (B) Halothane
   (C) Isoflurane
   (D) Nitrous oxide
   (E) None of the above

11. CNS toxicity of local anesthetics is thought to be due to

   (A) direct stimulation of seizure foci in the cerebral cortex

   (B) depression of the cardiovascular system

   (C) direct stimulation of excitation neurons in the cerebral cortex

   (D) depression of inhibitor fibers in the cerebral cortex, which leads to unopposed facilitory neurons

   (E) none of the above

12. Local anesthetic depression of myocardial contractility is most closely related to the

   (A) pKa of the drug
   (B) volume of drug injected
   (C) calcium channel blockade
   (D) potency of drug injected
   (E) site of injection

13. Per kilogram of body weight, the highest dose requirement for thiopental at induction is in

   (A) the elderly
   (B) 30- to 50-year-old adults
   (C) adolescents
   (D) 6- to 12-month-old infants
   (E) 1- to 6-month-old infants

14. Which of the following orders of speed of recovery and return of psychomotor function is correct?

   (A) Propofol > midazolam > thiopental > methohexital

   (B) Propofol > thiopental > midazolam > methohexital

   (C) Propofol > midazolam > methohexital > thiopental

   (D) Propofol > methohexital > thiopental > midazolam

   (E) Propofol > thiopental > methohexital > midazolam

15. True statements concerning *cis*-atracurium include all the following EXCEPT

(A) *cis*-atracurium is one of the 10 isomers of atracurium

(B) one of the breakdown products of *cis*-atracurium is laudanosine

(C) *cis*-atracurium elicits significant histamine release upon injection. Doses must be titrated to the patient's blood pressure

(D) *cis*-atracurium is metabolized by Hoffmann elimination and ester hydrolysis

(E) *cis*-atracurium is an improvement over atracurium because of its more stable hemodynamic profile in that there is much less histamine release

16. Which of the following induction agents would be likely to cause hypotension when used in a healthy 40-year-old man who has been NPO for 8 h?

(A) Thiopental 4 mg/kg
(B) Propofol 2.5 mg/kg
(C) Ketamine 2 mg/kg
(D) Etomidate 0.3 mg/kg
(E) None of the above

17. Administration of 1 mg/kg of succinylcholine (SCh) 5 min after 5 mg of neostigmine has been given will result in

(A) prolongation of effect of SCh for less than 5 min
(B) prolongation of effect of SCh for 10 to 40 min
(C) shortened duration of effect of SCh
(D) completely unpredictable effects
(E) none of the above

18. All the following statements concerning rocuronium are true EXCEPT

(A) rocuronium is an analog of vecuronium

(B) the onset of neuromuscular blockade of rocuronium occurs in 60 to 90 s, making it a possible substitute for succinylcholine in the rapid intubation of the trachea

(C) rocuronium maintains cardiac stability because it has only weak vagolytic properties and does not elicit the release of histamine

(D) rocuronium is metabolized by both hepatic and renal pathways

(E) there is an active metabolite of rocuronium that is 50 percent as potent as rocuronium

Directions: Each question below contains four suggested responses of which **one or more** is correct. Select:

(A)	if	**1, 2, and 3**	are correct
(B)	if	**1 and 3**	are correct
(C)	if	**2 and 4**	are correct
(D)	if	**4**	is correct
(E)	if	**1, 2, 3, and 4**	are correct

19. Causes of hypotension after large intravenous bolus doses of opioids include

    (1) reduction in sympathetic tone
    (2) stimulation of peripheral beta$_2$ receptors
    (3) histamine release and resultant venodilation
    (4) increase in renin-angiotensin levels

20. Possible mechanisms for changes in heart rate after administration of opioids include

    (1) stimulation of the central vagal tone
    (2) blockade of the central sympathetic nervous system
    (3) direct effect on both the sinoatrial and atrioventricular nodes
    (4) blockade of calcium channels

21. True statements concerning opioids and their effects on respiration include

    (1) the slope of the ventilatory response to CO_2 is decreased
    (2) minute ventilation responses to increases in CO_2 are shifted to the right
    (3) the apneic threshold is increased
    (4) opioids decrease hypoxic pulmonary vasoconstriction (HPV)

22. True statements concerning opioids and muscle rigidity include

    (1) opioid rigidity progresses in a temporal sequence involving first the extremities and last the abdomen and thorax
    (2) muscle rigidity is due to stimulation of acetylcholine receptor sites at the motor end plate, which causes depolarization
    (3) alfentanyl causes the lowest incidence of rigidity
    (4) rapid infusions of large volumes of opioids are most likely to cause rigidity

23. Concerning opioids and their effects on cerebral blood flow (CBF), cerebral metabolic rate (CMR), and intracranial pressure (ICP), true statements include

    (1) narcotic analgesics generally produce decreases in CMR and ICP
    (2) opioids cause cerebral vasoconstriction
    (3) autoregulation remains in response to increases in arterial CO_2, decreases in O_2, and changes in blood pressure
    (4) opioids cause a decrease in production of cerebral spinal fluid (CSF) and maintain absorption of CSF

24. Remifentanil may be attractive for use in the outpatient setting because

   (1) remifentanil has an extremely quick onset, similar to alfentanil
   (2) if given intraoperatively, remifentanil provides excellent long-term postoperative pain relief
   (3) the half-life of remifentanil is approximately 10 min
   (4) remifentanil also acts as an antiemetic

25. True statements regarding naloxone include that it

   (1) reverses biliary spasm secondary to opioids
   (2) inhibits histamine release that accompanies morphine administration
   (3) is primarily a μ receptor antagonist
   (4) has a longer duration of action than does naltrexone

26. Respiratory depression in the newborn may be caused by

   (1) 1 μg/kg fentanyl within 15 min of delivery
   (2) 100 mg meperidine more than 4 h before delivery
   (3) 50 mg meperidine within 1 h of delivery
   (4) 5 mg morphine within 2 h of delivery

27. Truncal skeletal muscle rigidity associated with opioid agonists is

   (1) increased in severity with rapid infusion and large bolus infusion
   (2) more commonly observed in elderly patients
   (3) found with the highest incidence with alfentanil
   (4) prevented or decreased by pretreatment with muscle relaxants

28. Opioid-induced nausea and vomiting is related to

   (1) direct stimulation of the chemoreceptor trigger zone in the floor of the fourth ventricle
   (2) direct stimulation of the vomiting center in the medulla
   (3) opioid's effect in delaying gastric emptying
   (4) an antagonistic effect at the dopamine receptors

29. Which of the following drugs may have drug interactions with opioid agonists?

   (1) Amphetamines
   (2) Monoamine oxidase inhibitors
   (3) Norepinephrine
   (4) Atropine

30. Which of the following maneuvers can be used to decrease the amount of inhalation anesthetic needed?

   (1) The addition of an opioid narcotic
   (2) The addition of muscle relaxants
   (3) Nerve block in the region of surgery
   (4) Hemodilution to hematocrit of 25

31. True statements include which of the following?

    (1)   Isoflurane increases resting Pa_{CO_2} more than enflurane does in spontaneously ventilated unstimulated patients

    (2)   The inhibitory effect of inhaled agents on ventilatory response to hypoxia is present only at 0.5 minimum alveolar concentration (MAC) or higher

    (3)   The depressant effect of inhaled agents on CO_2 response is completely eliminated with surgical stimulation

    (4)   Nitrous oxide at 50% has no effect on ventilatory responses to CO_2

32. With regard to uptake and distribution of inhaled anesthetics, true statements include

    (1)   the solubility of the following agents in decreasing order is desflurane > ether > halothane > enflurane > nitrous oxide

    (2)   an increase in cardiac output and ventilation affects the rate of anesthetic rise more with the least soluble agents and less with the more soluble agents

    (3)   ventilation-perfusion abnormalities affect the rate of anesthetic rise of more soluble agents and have little effect on that of the least soluble agents

    (4)   the concentration effect allows the acceleration of anesthetic uptake by increasing the inspired concentration

33. True statements regarding MAC include

    (1)   MAC is lower at high altitudes, where atmospheric pressure is lower

    (2)   MAC changes with age; it is maximal in late infancy

    (3)   the physical property of general anesthetics that correlates best with anesthetic potency is vapor pressure

    (4)   it is assumed that brain and alveolar concentrations are equal once equilibrium is reached

SUMMARY OF DIRECTIONS

A	B	C	D	E
1,2,3 only	1,3 only	2,4 only	4 only	All are correct

34. True statements regarding MAC include

(1) MAC is age-dependent
(2) the oil/gas partition coefficient is directly correlated with MAC
(3) MACs for inhaled agents may be considered as additive
(4) the following agents are correctly listed in descending order of MAC: halothane > enflurane > isoflurane > methoxyflurane > nitrous oxide

35. True statements include

(1) the depressant effect of the inhaled agents on mucociliary function may be a contributing factor toward the development of postoperative pulmonary complications
(2) isoflurane is the only inhalational agent with no effect on the baroreceptor function
(3) enflurane has more negative inotropic effect than does halothane
(4) inhaled agents increase the slope of the ventilatory response curve to CO_2

36. True statements regarding inhaled anesthetics include

(1) depression of ventilation (measured by elevated resting Pa_{CO_2}) occurs in the following order: enflurane > isoflurane > halothane
(2) halothane, isoflurane, and enflurane at clinical concentrations all depress the ventilatory response to hypoxia
(3) halothane, isoflurane, and enflurane all reduce mean arterial pressure; halothane and enflurane accomplish this primarily by reducing cardiac output while isoflurane does so by reducing systemic vascular resistance
(4) inhaled anesthetics are all direct depressants of myocardial contraction

37. Regarding the inhaled anesthetics halothane, isoflurane, and enflurane

(1) halothane increases cerebral blood flow the most, and enflurane the least
(2) uncoupling in the brain occurs and refers to the loss of autoregulation, such that perfusion pressure in the brain becomes unrelated to changes in vessel diameter
(3) halothane is metabolized the most, followed by isoflurane and then enflurane
(4) at 1.5 MAC of isoflurane, burst suppression appears on EEG; at 2.0 to 2.5 MAC of isoflurane, electrical silence appears

38. Regarding uptake of anesthetic gases, true statements include which of the following?

(1) During an induction with 3% halothane in oxygen, 1% isoflurane is suddenly substituted for the halothane; the second gas effect would apply to isoflurane—i.e., the presence of halothane in the alveoli would speed the rate of rise of the alveolar concentration of isoflurane

(2) The effect of increasing minute ventilation on speeding induction with anesthetic gases is greater for soluble than for insoluble agents

(3) A blood gas partition coefficient of 2.4, as in the case of halothane, means the partial pressure of halothane in the blood will be 2.4 times that in the gas phase when equilibrium is reached

(4) The curves below represent the rate of rise of alveolar concentration with time for several anesthetic gases; from top to bottom, the top four curves represent nitrous oxide, desflurane, isoflurane, and halothane

39. The fulminant form of halothane hepatitis

(1) does not affect children

(2) is an entity attributable to halothane exposure but probably is applicable to enflurane as well

(3) carries a good prognosis if detected early

(4) may be due to an oxidative metabolite of halothane

40. Complications of using nitrous oxide in a patient who is undergoing pneumoencephalography include

(1) an increase in ADH secretion

(2) potentiation of narcotics

(3) prolongation of nondepolarizing muscle relaxants

(4) an increase in intracranial pressure

41. True statements on nitrous oxide toxicity include

(1) it occurs only with chronic exposure

(2) it is related to inactivation of the enzyme methionine synthetase

(3) pretreatment with large doses of folinic acid can prevent bone marrow toxicity

(4) only the hematopoietic system is affected

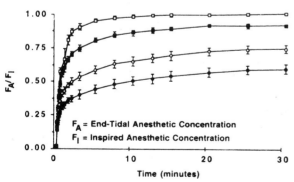

From Anaquest Prescribing Information and N. Yasuda, with permission.

42. Potential problems with the use of nitrous oxide (N_2O) include which of the following?

    (1) Use of 75% N_2O during a general anesthetic for which an endotracheal tube is used can result in a doubling or tripling of the size of the endotracheal tube cuff and subsequent excessive pressure on tracheal mucosa

    (2) N_2O reduces the cobalt in vitamin B_{12}, which causes inactivation of thymidine synthetase and the production of mutations in DNA

    (3) N_2O exposure has been associated with an increased incidence of spontaneous abortions in pregnant women but not with an increased incidence of birth defects

    (4) Unless supplemental oxygen is given after discontinuation of 70% N_2O, diffusion hypoxia may occur because N_2O is five times as soluble as nitrogen in blood

43. The current recommendations with respect to patients on monoamine oxidase (MAO) inhibitors include

    (1) they should have their medications discontinued for at least 2 weeks preoperatively because of the cardiovascular instability that can occur in the perioperative period

    (2) hyperpyrexic coma is a risk with the use of narcotics

    (3) much larger doses of the direct α and β agonists are needed because of their decreased receptor sensitivity

    (4) cocaine, ephedrine, and meperidine are all drugs that should be avoided

44. Which of the following inhaled anesthetics will produce inorganic F^- (dichloroacetic acid) when metabolized?

    (1) Isoflurane
    (2) Enflurane
    (3) Desflurane
    (4) Methoxyflurane

45. Inhaled agents that are potentially nephrotoxic through production of inorganic F^- include

    (1) sevoflurane
    (2) halothane
    (3) isoflurane
    (4) methoxyflurane

46. Preoperative administration of a single oral dose of clonidine 4 to 5 μg per kilogram body weight to a patient who will undergo major vascular surgery will

    (1) lower basal heart rate
    (2) blunt the sympathetic nervous system response to intubation
    (3) decrease the intraoperative requirements for inhaled agents and narcotics
    (4) reduce intraoperative fluctuations of heart rate and blood pressure

47. True statements about nitroprusside include which of the following?

(1) In most instances, the first sign of nitroprusside toxicity in a patient under general anesthesia is hypoxemia

(2) In nitroprusside-induced toxicity, the venous blood P_{O_2} may be abnormally high

(3) It has less chance of causing toxicity than does nitroglycerin

(4) The recommended dose for acute administration is approximately 1.5 mg/kg

48. Drugs and their mechanisms of action are correctly described in which of the following statements?

(1) Digoxin inhibits myocardial cell calcium pumps, which causes increased intracellular calcium and improved contractility

(2) Warfarin (Coumadin) interferes with the action of hydroxylase in the conversion of factors 2, 7, 9, and 10

(3) Heparin combines with thromboplastin and inhibits the conversion of prothrombin to thrombin and fibrinogen to fibrin

(4) Oral hypoglycemics stimulate insulin release by pancreatic beta cells

49. True statements about drugs and their effects include which of the following?

(1) Phenothiazines work by enhancing dopaminergic pathways, thereby improving the patient's mood

(2) Of the three calcium channel blockers, verapamil has the smallest negative inotropic effect, diltiazem has the greatest antihypertensive effect, and nifedipine has the greatest effect on heart rate

(3) Aminophylline, by inhibiting phosphodiesterase and the breakdown of cyclic AMP, protects against halothane-induced dysrhythmias

(4) Tricyclic antidepressants block reuptake of norepinephrine, have anticholinergic effects, and may produce exaggerated hypertensive responses in the presence of direct-acting pressors

50. In performing intravenous sympathetic regional blockade,

(1) guanethidine will give 3 days of dystrophic pain relief

(2) reserpine can result in postural hypotension from circulating drug

(3) a mixture of bretylium and lidocaine can result in a 20-day block of pain

(4) stellate ganglion block with bupivacaine lasts longer than any of the above

51. The problems associated with the use of nonselective beta-antagonist therapy include

(1) bronchospasm
(2) cardiac failure
(3) masking of the symptoms and signs of hypoglycemia
(4) drug interactions with calcium channel blockers

52. True statements about local anesthetics and their actions include

(1) the most important factor governing the duration of action of a local anesthetic is pKa
(2) ester local anesthetics have higher pKa's than do the amides, which means that at physiologic pH there is more ionized form of the ester drug than of the amide drug
(3) addition of vasoconstrictor agents, such as epinephrine, to local anesthetic solutions usually increases the peak plasma concentrations of local anesthetics
(4) the pKa of a local anesthetic is the pH at which the drug is half ionized and half un-ionized

53. Mixtures of two different local anesthetics

(1) may cause the metabolites of one drug to interfere with the action of another
(2) minimize toxicity
(3) may result in slower onset and briefer duration of action
(4) can combine the features of rapid onset and long duration

54. Nitroglycerin, which is used chiefly in the treatment of angina pectoris,

(1) acts primarily on venous capacitance vessels
(2) prevents angina in patients with atherosclerotic heart disease by increasing coronary blood flow
(3) decreases esophageal muscle tone
(4) produces an increase in bleeding time by decreasing platelet aggregation

55. Which of the following is true?

(1) *p*-Aminobenzoic acid is often the antigen that provokes the allergic reaction to ester local anesthetics
(2) Procaine can cause methemoglobinemia, which usually requires no treatment but can be successfully treated with methylene blue
(3) Neurotoxicity related to 2-chloroprocaine was attributed to the low pH of the preservative that had been included in the solution
(4) Na bisulfite was previously included as a preservative in many local anesthetic solutions and might have accounted for some of the allergic reactions related to the amide local anesthetics

56. Epinephrine added to a local anesthetic solution will

(1) increase the duration of local anesthetic action
(2) reduce the risk of developing systemic toxicity
(3) deepen sensory blockade
(4) work via local vasoconstriction and central α adrenoceptor stimulation

57. True statements about local anesthetics include which of the following?

(1) The ratio of doses required to cause cardiac compared with central nervous system toxicity is higher for lidocaine than for bupivacaine

(2) Etidocaine is unsuitable for epidural anesthesia for labor because at the concentration required for adequate sensory blockade, motor blockade is profound

(3) Prilocaine has less chance of causing systemic central nervous system or cardiac toxicity than do other local anesthetics, but it may cause methemoglobinemia

(4) Tetracaine is an excellent topical anesthetic for the airways, but the combination of rapid absorption and high toxicity makes it more dangerous than lidocaine to use by this route

58. When epinephrine is added to anesthetic solutions, it

(1) prolongs the block of all agents when they are used for epidural anesthesia

(2) is especially effective in prolonging the block of highly lipid-soluble agents

(3) is far superior to all other vasoconstrictors in prolonging blockade

(4) prolongs the block of all agents when they are used for local infiltration

SUMMARY OF DIRECTIONS

A	B	C	D	E
1,2,3 only	1,3 only	2,4 only	4 only	All are correct

59. Which of the following statement(s) about the use of local anesthetic is true?

    (1) Plasma concentrations of lidocaine can become elevated in patients with poor cardiac or liver function
    (2) Duration of action of lidocaine is more prolonged in the elderly
    (3) Lidocaine elimination is prolonged in neonates as a result of the immaturity of the hepatic enzymes that metabolize these local anesthetics
    (4) Continuous infusion rate of bupivacaine in neonates needs to be higher than in adults because the pharmacokinetic profile for bupivacaine is different in newborns

60. Which of the following mechanisms may account for the increased CNS toxicity observed with respiratory acidosis?

    (1) Increased Pa_{CO_2} increases cerebral blood flow
    (2) Increased protein binding leads to increased CNS drug concentration
    (3) Intracellular acidosis leads to ion trapping of the active cationic form of the local anesthetic
    (4) Increased cationic form of the local anesthetic increases the diffusion of the drug into CNS

61. Local anesthetics have direct cardiotoxic effects, including

    (1) negative inotropic action on cardiac tissue
    (2) prolonged conduction time through the heart
    (3) depression of the rapid phase of depolarization
    (4) decrease in duration of action potential

62. Correct statements concerning bupivacaine cardiotoxicity include that it

    (1) is enhanced by acidosis and hypoxia
    (2) may result in reentrant dysrhythmias
    (3) may be due to high myocardial uptake of the drug
    (4) is characterized by the formation of methemoglobin

63. Ropivacaine, in comparison with bupivacaine,

    (1) is slightly less potent in vivo
    (2) has the same duration of action
    (3) has less cardiac toxicity
    (4) is cleared less rapidly from the circulation

64. A patient reports that he experienced prolonged paralysis after administration of succinylcholine during prior anesthesia. Which of the following drugs might produce a prolonged toxic effect in this patient if he is given an overdose?

    (1) Mepivacaine
    (2) Bupivacaine
    (3) Etidocaine
    (4) Tetracaine

65. True statements about local anesthetics include which of the following?

    (1)   The ester or amide linkage has no effect on the potency of a local anesthetic

    (2)   Potency of local anesthetics is enhanced by the addition of alkyl groups

    (3)   There is a strong correlation between potency of local anesthetics in vivo and in vitro

    (4)   The hydrophobic nature of a local anesthetic is an important determinant of its potency

66. Onset of action of local anesthetics is dependent on

    (1)   lipid solubility of the drug

    (2)   pKa of the drug

    (3)   potency of the drug

    (4)   concentration of drug injection

67. Duration of local anesthetic blockade can be influenced by

    (1)   the pKa of the drug

    (2)   the rate of onset of drug action

    (3)   whether the drug is an amide or an ester type

    (4)   the effects of the drug on blood vessels in the vicinity of the injection site

68. Sodium bicarbonate added to certain local anesthetics will

    (1)   enhance the depth of sensory blockade

    (2)   increase the duration of the block

    (3)   enhance the depth of motor blockade

    (4)   lessen the onset time of the block

69. The dose of local anesthetics during pregnancy needs to be reduced

    (1)   only during the third trimester

    (2)   depending on the specific local anesthetic to be administered

    (3)   only when the drug is used for central neural axis blockade because of the anatomic considerations during pregnancy

    (4)   throughout the pregnancy because the sensitivity to local anesthetics is increased during pregnancy

70. True statements regarding methohexital include that it

    (1)   has a greater hepatic clearance than does thiopental

    (2)   is more potent than thiopental

    (3)   results in more rapid recovery than does thiopental

    (4)   has been associated with seizures in high doses

71. Droperidol is correctly characterized by which of the following statements?

    (1)   It is a dopaminergic receptor antagonist

    (2)   It has antagonist effects at peripheral alpha-adrenergic receptors

    (3)   It has no effect on resting ventilation and CO_2 responsiveness

    (4)   It should be avoided in patients with pheochromocytoma because of reported extreme hypertension associated with its use in these patients

72. True statement(s) regarding droperidol include that it

   (1)   works by decreasing the action of dopamine at postsynaptic receptors

   (2)   is effective in treating motion sickness

   (3)   decreases blood pressure secondary to alpha blockade

   (4)   alters the ventilatory response to carbon dioxide

73. Ketamine affects the respiratory system in which of the following ways?

   (1)   Ketamine has minimal effect on central respiratory drive

   (2)   Ketamine is a bronchial smooth muscle relaxant

   (3)   Swallow, cough, sneeze, and gag reflexes are relatively intact after administration of ketamine

   (4)   Ketamine is an excellent antisialagogue

74. True statement(s) about ketamine include that it

   (1)   is metabolized extensively by hepatic microsomal enzymes

   (2)   has increased metabolism and diminished drug effect when used with halothane or diazepam

   (3)   is a phencyclidine derivative that produces "dissociative anesthesia"

   (4)   has poor analgesic properties

75. Side effects associated with etomidate include

   (1)   high incidence of nausea and vomiting

   (2)   adrenal suppression lasting at least 6 h

   (3)   enhanced neuromuscular blockade with nondepolarizing muscle relaxants

   (4)   triggering of porphyria in susceptible individuals

76. Properties of etomidate include that it

(1) maintains hemodynamic stability
(2) causes minimal respiratory depression
(3) affords cerebral protection
(4) alters hepatic function

77. Etomidate may be useful in neurosurgical cases for which of the following reasons?

(1) Etomidate lowers intracranial pressure (ICP), cerebral blood flow (CBF), and cerebral metabolic rate ($CMRO_2$) without altering mean arterial pressure
(2) Etomidate is antiepileptogenic
(3) Etomidate maintains cerebral autoregulation
(4) Etomidate ablates brainstem evoked potentials and thus causes a decrease in latency and increased amplitude

78. True statement(s) concerning propofol include

(1) propofol is insoluble in water
(2) propofol is rapidly metabolized by the liver
(3) the clearance of propofol exceeds hepatic blood flow
(4) propofol has prolonged clearance in patients with renal failure

79. True statements concerning propofol and its effects on the cardiovascular system include that it

(1) causes a decrease in venous return to the right heart
(2) decreases myocardial contractility
(3) decreases afterload
(4) sensitizes the heart to dysrhythmias

80. Propofol is accurately characterized by which of the following statements?

(1) Propofol is an antianalgesic similar to barbiturates
(2) Propofol commonly causes postoperative agitation that results in prolonged stays in the recovery room
(3) Propofol causes increases in intracranial pressure (ICP) and intraocular pressure (IOP)
(4) Propofol causes respiratory and cardiovascular depression

81. Side effects of propofol include

(1) potentiation of neuromuscular blockade
(2) triggering of malignant hyperthermia (MH)
(3) adrenal suppression of cortisol release
(4) significant antiemetic properties

82. True statements on the pharmacokinetics of propofol include

(1) there are no significant differences between men and women in the pharmacokinetics of propofol
(2) clearance and central volume are both increased in children
(3) renal diseases decrease its clearance, while hepatic diseases have no significant effect
(4) clearance and central volume of distribution are both decreased in the elderly

83. With respect to the action and pharmacokinetics of thiopental,

(1) GABA receptor stimulation is the most likely cause of sedative effects
(2) the short duration of sleep is due to redistribution of drug
(3) sleep is rapidly induced because of high perfusion of the brain
(4) in the usual clinical doses, obese patients have a longer sleep time because of high affinity for fat

84. True statements about barbiturates include

(1) the predominant cardiovascular effect of thiopental and methohexital is depression of cardiac contractility
(2) injection of thiopental into an artery of an arm can result in joint inflammation of the fingers and Raynaud's phenomenon
(3) in a dose-related manner, thiopental initially produces on EEG a progression to alpha and beta activity, followed by burst suppression and eventually a flat EEG
(4) if barbiturates are given to patients with acute intermittent or variegate porphyria, paralysis and death may occur

85. The effects of barbiturates on the respiratory system include

(1) decreases in the rate and depth of breathing until apnea occurs
(2) bronchodilation and depressed laryngeal reflexes
(3) decreased response to hypercarbia and hypoxemia
(4) significant salivation

86. True statements concerning barbiturates and their effects on the central nervous system include which of the following?

(1) Thiopental produces dose-related depression of the electroencephalogram (EEG) from the awake alpha patterns to burst suppression and a flat EEG
(2) Barbiturates decrease cerebral metabolic rate ($CMRO_2$), cerebral blood flow (CBF), and intracranial pressure (ICP), but cerebral perfusion pressure (CCP) is maintained
(3) Barbiturates decrease intraocular pressure (IOP)
(4) Thiopental grossly alters somatosensory evoked potentials by increasing latency and decreasing amplitudes

87. Concerning barbiturates and their effect on the cardiovascular system, true statements include which of the following?

(1) Barbiturates sensitize the heart to dysrhythmia even with normoxia and normocarbia
(2) Barbiturates induce venodilation and decrease myocardial contractility
(3) Barbiturates increase sympathetic outflow from the CNS
(4) An induction dose of barbiturates increases heart rate via baroreceptor reflexes in response to a decrease in cardiac output

88. True statements about benzodiazepines include which of the following?

    (1) Midazolam and diazepam have the same volume of distribution, but the elimination half-life of diazepam is more than 10 times as long

    (2) The main hemodynamic effect of midazolam is a reduction in systemic vascular resistance

    (3) The combination of opioids and benzodiazepines can have synergistic hemodynamic effects; that is, the decrease in blood pressure seen with the combination can be much greater than that seen with either drug alone

    (4) The biggest hazard with midazolam administration is respiratory depression

89. Flumazenil is accurately characterized by which of the following descriptions?

    (1) Flumazenil produces reversal of the unconsciousness, respiratory depression, sedation, and amnesia caused by benzodiazepines

    (2) Flumazenil competes with benzodiazepines at the benzodiazepine receptor site

    (3) Flumazenil has intrinsic benzodiazepine-receptor agonist effects

    (4) Flumazenil normally causes significant stimulation of the sympathetic system

90. With respect to the pharmacokinetics of benzodiazepines,

    (1) age is a significant factor in the clearance of diazepam

    (2) obesity does not alter the clearance of lorazepam

    (3) induction dose of midazolam should be based on total body weight

    (4) infusion of midazolam should be based on lean body weight

SUMMARY OF DIRECTIONS

A	B	C	D	E
1,2,3 only	1,3 only	2,4 only	4 only	All are correct

91. Correct statements about succinylcholine would include which of the following?

    (1) Significant hyperkalemia can occur after succinylcholine is given in all the following conditions: burn injury, muscular dystrophy, upper motor neuron diseases, and spinal cord transection

    (2) Administration of a small dose of a nondepolarizing muscle relaxant several minutes before succinylcholine is an effective means of preventing postoperative myalgias

    (3) Bradydysrhythmias are commonly seen after a second dose

    (4) A defasciculating dose of nondepolarizing muscle relaxant before succinylcholine administration has been shown to effectively and reliably prevent succinylcholine-induced intraocular pressures

92. Pseudocholinesterase level is reduced in

    (1) pregnancy
    (2) liver disease
    (3) patients on cytotoxic drugs
    (4) patients with a dibucaine number of 20

93. Which of the following muscle relaxants will cause the release of histamine?

    (1) Atracurium
    (2) Curare
    (3) Metocurine
    (4) Vecuronium

94. In regard to muscle relaxants, burn patients

    (1) can safely receive succinylcholine (SCh) within the first few hours of a burn

    (2) should not receive SCh as long as infection is present

    (3) show relative resistance to nondepolarizing muscle relaxants

    (4) will show a hyperkalemic response to SCh that depends on the dose of SCh and the extent of the burn

95. Succinylcholine (SCh) should be avoided in patients with

    (1) hyperkalemia
    (2) burn injuries affecting less than 20 percent of total body surface area
    (3) hemiplegia
    (4) cerebral palsy

96. True statements about succinylcholine include

    (1) the termination of action of succinylcholine is due to rapid hydrolysis by pseudocholinesterase at the motor end plate

    (2) a dibucaine number of 80 indicates 80 percent inhibition of pseudocholinesterase by dibucaine

    (3) since there is no way to monitor for a phase II desensitization block, it is recommended that succinylcholine not be given by continuous infusion

    (4) succinylcholine may have a prolonged relaxant effect if given after reversal of a nondepolarizing block because neostigmine antagonizes pseudocholinesterase

97. Which of the following would prolong or enhance the effect of succinylcholine (SCh)?

(1) Neostigmine
(2) Quinidine
(3) Magnesium
(4) Pyridostigmine

98. Factors affecting reversal of a nondepolarizing neuromuscular blockade include which of the following?

(1) Pa_{CO_2} with the range of 20 to 30 torr will not affect the ability to reverse neuromuscular blockade
(2) All the following are muscarinic side effects of anticholinesterase drugs: slowing of heart rate, bronchoconstriction, and bronchial secretion production
(3) Metabolic acidosis, but not alkalosis, will prevent antagonism of a nondepolarizing block by neostigmine
(4) All the following can potentiate a nondepolarizing neuromuscular block: gentamycin, clindamycin, magnesium, and quinidine

99. True statements include which of the following?

(1) Pharmacokinetics and pharmacodynamics of vecuronium for neonates and infants are different from those for adults
(2) Hypothermia shortens the action of atracurium
(3) Adults and neonates have similar durations of action for atracurium
(4) The dose of anticholinsterase inhibitors should be reduced in patients with renal failure

100. Which of the following drugs may prolong the action of nondepolarizing muscle relaxants?

(1) Tetracycline
(2) Furosemide
(3) Streptomycin
(4) Phenytoin

101. True statements include which of the following?

(1) Tachycardia induced by pancuronium is secondary to pancuronium's inhibition of catecholamine reuptake, ganglionic stimulation, and vagolytic effects
(2) Enflurane, halothane, isoflurane, and desflurane all augment the effects of nondepolarizing muscle relaxants
(3) Vecuronium is devoid of autonomic effects
(4) Atracurium should not be used in patients with epilepsy because of the CNS stimulatory effects of its metabolite laudanosine

102. True statements include

(1) if serum potassium is normal, succinylcholine may be used in patients with renal failure
(2) the elimination of vecuronium, metocurine, and gallamine is equally affected in renal failure
(3) patients with liver failure require a larger initial dose and less frequent "top off" of pancuronium
(4) the elimination half-life and duration of action of atracurium are prolonged in patients with cirrhosis

103. With regard to the augmentation effect of inhaled anesthetics on muscle relaxants, true statements include

    (1)   it is dose-dependent for desflurane and halothane but not for isoflurane and enflurane

    (2)   inhaled anesthetics reduce ionic conductance through nicotinic receptors

    (3)   a *d*-tubocurarine neuromuscular block is less likely to be affected by inhaled anesthetics than is one produced by vecuronium or rocuronium

    (4)   the mechanism for isoflurane is partly related to isoflurane's enhancement of blood flow to muscle

104. Extrajunctional receptors in the neuromuscular junction are found in the muscle of

    (1)   stroke patients
    (2)   bedridden patients
    (3)   patients with spinal cord injuries
    (4)   patients under age 2

SUMMARY OF DIRECTIONS

A	B	C	D	E
1,2,3	1,3	2,4	4	All are
only	only	only	only	correct

105. Cholinesterase inhibitors with effects on the central nervous system include

   (1) neostigmine
   (2) edrophonium
   (3) pyridostigmine
   (4) physostigmine

106. Edrophonium is accurately characterized by which of the following statements?

   (1) It produces irreversible inhibition of acetylcholinesterase
   (2) It produces carbamyl esters to inhibit acetylcholinesterase
   (3) It is intermediate in onset of action compared with neostigmine and pyridostigmine
   (4) It is eliminated primarily via the kidneys

107. True comparisons between glycopyrrolate and atropine and scopolamine include that glycopyrrolate

   (1) is poorly lipid-soluble compared with atropine and scopolamine
   (2) crosses the placenta more easily than does atropine
   (3) is a less potent antisialagogue than scopolamine
   (4) is intermediate in its effects on pupillary size between atropine and scopolamine

108. Regarding neuromuscular transmission,

   (1) muscle relaxants bind to the same site on the acetylcholine receptor as does acetylcholine; whether channel blockade or transmission occurs depends on competitive interaction between molecules of acetylcholine and muscle relaxants
   (2) two molecules of acetylcholine must be bound to an acetylcholine receptor to open its ion channel; one molecule of antagonist (muscle relaxant) is required to keep it closed
   (3) denervated muscle cells develop extrajunctional receptors, which are less sensitive to nondepolarizing muscle relaxants than are junctional receptors
   (4) the reason succinylcholine has a longer duration of action than does acetylcholine is that pseudocholinesterase metabolizes succinylcholine more slowly than acetylcholinesterase metabolizes acetylcholine

109. Correct statements about neuromuscular transmission include which of the following?

(1) Calcium channel blockers (nifedipine, verapamil, diltiazem) can have profound effects on neuromuscular transmission

(2) When acetylcholine reacts with the nicotinic acetylcholine receptor, a channel opens and sodium and calcium flow into the muscle cell while potassium flows out

(3) Acetylcholine molecules that are released into the synaptic cleft and do not bind instantly with acetylcholine receptors diffuse into the bloodstream, where they are promptly metabolized by acetylcholinesterase

(4) The acetylcholine receptor is a protein; acetylcholine binds to two areas on this protein known as *alpha subunits*

110. Anticholinesterases (e.g., edrophonium) have muscarinic as well as nicotinic effects. Some of the muscarinic effects include

(1) miosis

(2) stimulation of autonomic ganglia

(3) bronchoconstriction

(4) decreased bladder and increased sphincter tone

111. Which of the following nondepolarizing muscle relaxants may be classified as a benzylisoquinoline?

(1) Metocurine

(2) Atracurium

(3) *d*-Tubocurarine

(4) Vecuronium

112. True statements about neuromuscular blockade include which of the following?

(1) Seventy-five to eighty percent of muscle end-plate acetylcholine receptors may still be blocked in a patient who has received a nondepolarizing muscle relaxant but has normal tidal volume breathing

(2) After neuromuscular blockade with a nondepolarizing muscle relaxant, head lift for 5 s can be achieved; 33 percent of muscle end-plate acetylcholine receptors may still be blocked

(3) Sustained tetanus at 100 Hz is a more sensitive indicator of muscle relaxant reversal than is a train-of-four without fade

(4) Simultaneous stimulation of the diaphragm and the ulnar nerve with equal current reveals that the diaphragm is more resistant to nondepolarizing muscle relaxants than is the ulnar nerve

113. True statements about drugs and their effects on the autonomic nervous system include which of the following?

(1) Atropine may precipitate bronchospasm

(2) The ganglionic blockade produced by trimethaphan refers to sympathetic ganglion blockade; the parasympathetic nervous system is not affected

(3) Ephedrine is a catecholamine

(4) Norepinephrine is a more potent venoconstrictor than is epinephrine, dopamine, ephedrine, or phenylephrine

114. True statements about the autonomic nervous system include

(1) the sympathetic and parasympathetic nervous systems differ in that preganglionic fibers of the parasympathetic nervous system are short compared with those of the sympathetic nervous system

(2) preganglionic sympathetic nervous system fibers liberate acetylcholine, which acts on nicotinic receptors

(3) a single sensory dermatome receives sympathetic innervation from spinal nerves at a single spinal level

(4) the celiac ganglion is a sympathetic nervous system structure that is innervated by T5–T12 and that innervates, among other structures, the kidneys

115. The effects of ganglionic blockade include

(1) vasodilation
(2) increased cardiac output
(3) tachycardia
(4) miosis

116. Concerning beta antagonistic drugs,

(1) metoprolol and atenolol are $beta_1$ selective

(2) the short half-life of esmolol is due primarily to its high lipid solubility

(3) there are marked differences in plasma levels between equal doses of oral and parenterally administered drugs

(4) as a group, they are primarily excreted by the kidney

SUMMARY OF DIRECTIONS

A	B	C	D	E
1,2,3 only	1,3 only	2,4 only	4 only	All are correct

117. The density of beta receptors can be influenced by

(1) continuous agonist stimulation
(2) continuous antagonist administration
(3) hyperthyroidism
(4) long-standing diabetes mellitus

118. True statements concerning adrenergic agents include

(1) dopamine has both direct and indirect receptor effects
(2) epinephrine has only direct receptor effects
(3) norepinephrine has virtually no beta$_2$ effects
(4) ephedrine has only direct receptor effects

119. True statements about angiotensin converting enzyme (ACE) inhibitors and the renin-angiotensin system include

(1) angiotensin converting enzyme is located predominantly in the kidney
(2) angioedema may occur after a single dose of any of the ACE inhibitors
(3) in patients on beta blockers, the addition of an ACE inhibitor may lead to complete heart block
(4) ACE inhibitors may cause renal failure

120. Problems associated with the use of beta blockade include

(1) the potential for drug-induced hypoglycemia
(2) effects on metabolism of other drugs
(3) increased incidence of laryngospasm
(4) increased risk of heart block when calcium channel blockers are used simultaneously

121. Potential benefits concerning the use of *cis*-atracurium in patients with hepatic failure include which of the following?

(1) *Cis*-atracurium is not dependent on hepatic or renal elimination
(2) *Cis*-atracurium has a more stable hemodynamic profile than does atracurium
(3) *Cis*-atracurium does not elicit histamine release
(4) *Cis*-atracurium is metabolized by Hoffmann elimination and ester hydrolysis

122. True statements regarding mannitol include that it

(1) is sugar that is not metabolized
(2) is reabsorbed from the renal tubules, which accounts for its long plasma half-life
(3) initially increases plasma volume before diuresis
(4) is associated with a high incidence of venous thrombosis

123. Verapamil is accurately described by which of the following statements?

(1) It is useful in conjunction with dantrolene in treating malignant hyperthermia
(2) It has local anesthetic activity
(3) It has greater effects on vascular smooth muscle than does nifedipine
(4) It potentiates the effects of nondepolarizing muscle relaxants

124. True statements regarding digoxin include

(1) it exerts its positive inotropic effect by inhibition of the sodium pump
(2) it causes increased parasympathetic nervous system activity
(3) excretion is primarily via the kidney with half-life prolonged in renal failure
(4) it is extensively metabolized in the liver to active metabolites

125. Amrinone is correctly characterized by which of the following statements?

(1) It is a synthetic catecholamine derived from tyrosine
(2) It produces dose-dependent increases in cardiac output and decreases in left ventricular end-diastolic pressure (LVEDP)
(3) Dosage should be lowered in a patient on digoxin because of synergistic toxicities
(4) It has side effects that include thrombocytopenia with prolonged use

126. True statements regarding furosemide include that it

(1) acts primarily in the medullary portion of the loop of Henle
(2) augments blockade by nondepolarizing muscle relaxants
(3) depletes myocardial potassium
(4) results in decreased plasma lithium levels

127. Which of the following antihypersensitive drugs may reduce anesthetic requirements in patients receiving a general anesthetic?

(1) Alpha-methyldopa
(2) Guanethidine
(3) Clonidine
(4) Captopril

128. The administration of captopril results in

(1) decreased plasma levels of angiotensin I
(2) slightly increased serum potassium
(3) decreased plasma levels of renin
(4) decreased levels of aldosterone

PHARMACOLOGY

ANSWERS

1. **The answer is C.** (Stoelting, *Anesthesia and Co-Existing Disease,* 3/e. p 239.) A Cheyne-Stokes respiratory pattern consists of periods of increasing hyperventilation alternating with apnea. The rate of ventilation increases markedly and then declines until apnea occurs. This pattern repeats in a rhythmic fashion. Cheyne-Stokes respiration usually occurs after a cerebral anoxic event and reflects brain damage. Opioids do not cause this respiratory pattern.

2. **The answer is E.** (Miller, 4/e. pp 326–327.) An increased clearance with a decreased volume of distribution will decrease the half-life of any opioid, and therefore, all the opioid's properties will be of shorter duration, including respiratory depression. When opioids are combined with any other respiratory depressant, the effects are synergistic. In addition, the magnitude of respiratory depression will increase with bolus injections of narcotics, increased age, and decreased hepatic blood flow.

3. **The answer is E.** (Miller, 4/e. pp 326–327.) During stress there is liberation of catabolic hormones from the neuroendocrine system—i.e., corticosteroids, catechoclamines, growth hormones, ACTH, prolactin, glucagon, thyroxine, and ADH—with a concomitant decrease of anabolic hormones. It originally was thought that the increase in levels of these hormones was necessary to improve survival during stress. The opposite is actually true. These hormones promote catabolism and lead to cardiovascular and hemodynamic instability. Narcotics may diminish this response to stress by blunting this neuroendocrine response. The exact mechanism by which opioids attenuate the stress response is not totally known but may be multifactorial.

4. **The answer is C.** (Miller, 4/e. pp 1334, 1337.) Opioids affect SSEPs minimally. Bolus administration sometimes may increase latency and decrease amplitude. This is less likely to occur when continuous infusions of opioids are used. Meperidine has minimal effect on SSEPs. Brainstem auditory evoked potentials are minimally affected by opioids or any kind

of anesthetic or combination thereof. Visual evoked potentials are affected by every type of anesthetic, including opioids, with increases in latency and decreases in amplitude.

5. **The answer is B.** (Miller, 4/e. pp 333, 335–337, 342–343.) Innovar is a combination of droperidol and fentanyl. Droperidol interrupts dopaminergic pathways in the brain and may exacerbate symptoms in patients with Parkinson's disease. Continuous infusion provides more analgesia in the immediate postoperative period. There also appears to be more hemodynamic stability and more rapid return to consciousness than with intermittent boluses.

6. **The answer is A.** (Miller, 4/e. pp 352–353.) Meperidine elicits greater histamine release than do the other opioids. Both in vitro and in vivo studies have shown that meperidine can be a potent negative inotrope compared with equal analgesic doses of all other narcotics. All other opioids will cause a decrease in heart rate, while meperidine will cause an increase in heart rate, via a direct effect, because of its structural similarity to atropine. In addition, heart rate may increase through a central toxic effect.

7. **The answer is A.** (Miller, 4/e. pp 345–346.) Remifentanil is a new ultra-short-acting μ receptor narcotic. It is not dependent on hepatic or renal metabolism. It is metabolized by nonspecific plasma and tissue esterases. Its onset is as quick as that of alfentanil. Remifentanil has a half-life of 10 min. It has all the usual side effects of opioids, which occur in a dose-dependent fashion: respiratory depression, chest wall rigidity, pruritis, and nausea and vomiting. Remifentanil does not cause histamine release and causes bradycardia, giving it a stable hemodynamic profile like that of its analog, fentanyl.

8. **The answer is D.** (Miller, 4/e. pp 353–357, 315–318.) In addition to the side effects listed, stroke and malignant dysrhythmias have occurred. Naloxone should be carefully titrated to avoid these complications and is best avoided in patients with cardiovascular and cerebrovascular disease. Clearance of alfentanil is lower than that of other opioids. The short duration of action is due to its small volume of distribution (which limits accumulation of drug in tissues), adequate lipid solubility (which allows brain penetration), and high degree of un-ionized drug (which also aids brain penetration).

9. **The answer is B.** (Miller, 4/e. pp 169–172.) Decreases in cardiac output with resultant decreases in renal blood flow are caused by all potent inhaled agents which lead to decreased renal function. In addition, direct metabolism of potent inhaled agents by the liver may produce levels of inorganic fluoride (F^-) which may potentially be nephrotoxic. The order of greatest level of metabolism to least is as follows: methoxyflurane > halothane > sevoflurane > enflurane > desflurane. Desflurane is minimally metabolized, 0.2 percent, such that nephrotoxic levels of F^- can never be attained.

10. **The answer is E.** (Miller, 4/e. pp 176–179.) No inhaled agents have been shown to be mutagenic in humans. Halothane and nitrous oxide have been found to be weakly mutagenic in in vitro testing.

11. **The answer is D.** (Miller, 4/e. pp 510–511.) There is no direct stimulation by local anesthetics of seizure foci or excitatory neurons. CNS toxic effects precede cardiovascular depression. Toxic effects in the CNS are excitatory in nature and are thought to be due to initial depression of inhibitory fibers. Twitching, tremors, and seizures are the signs of unopposed facilitory neurons at work. At higher tissue concentrations, neurons are also inhibited, leading to generalized CNS depression or coma.

12. **The answer is D.** (Miller, 4/e. pp 511–512.) Impairment of contractility is directly related to drug potency. It takes only a small dose of a potent drug, such as bupivacaine, to cause myocardial depression compared with the less potent drugs, such as chloroprocaine. However, a high enough dose or large enough volume of any local anesthetic, regardless of potency, can reduce cardiac contractility.

13. **The answer is E.** (Miller, 4/e. pp 234–235.) The highest dose requirement for thiopental at induction is in 1- to 6-month-old infants. The ED_{50} (the dose at which 50 percent of children are induced) at this age was found to be close to 7 mg/kg. In adults the induction dose range is 2.5 to 4.5 mg/kg, while in older children it is 5 to 6 mg/kg.

14. **The answer is D.** (Miller, 4/e. pp 2228–2229.) Propofol has the most rapid recovery of the four induction agents, irrespective of the maintenance agent. Methohexital has a slightly faster recovery than does thiopental. Barbiturates have more rapid recovery than do benzodiazepines such as midazolam.

15. **The answer is C.** (Miller, 4/e. pp 451–453.) *Cis*-atracurium is one of the 10 stereoisomers that compose atracurium. *Cis*-atracurium is an improvement over atracurium because there are minimal cardiovascular side effects, i.e., no changes in heart rate or blood pressure. *Cis*-atracurium does not elicit increases in plasma histamine levels upon administration. The metabolism of *cis*-atracurium is by Hoffmann elimination and ester hydrolysis. Laudanosine is a breakdown product, but the concentrations achieved are not clinically significant.

16. **The answer is B.** (Miller, 4/e. pp 238, 254, 262, 271–272.) In a healthy man who is euvolemic, 4 mg/kg is an induction dose of thiopental that should cause no significant changes in hemodynamics. Thiopental's predominant cardiovascular effect is venodilation, with some myocardial depressant effect that causes a decrease in cardiac output. However, the depressant effect of thiopental is minimized in a healthy person because heart rate also increases secondary to the only slightly affected baroreflex mechanism. No change in systemic vascular resistance occurs; therefore, no significant change in blood pressure occurs. The usual induction dose of ketamine is 2 mg/kg. Because of its sympathomimetic effect, ketamine increases systemic vascular resistance and heart rate and thus causes an increase in blood pressure. Propofol at 2.5 mg/kg, the usual induction dose, can cause a 25 to 40 percent decrease in blood pressure secondary to decreases in systemic vascular resistance and myocardial depressant effects. Etomidate at that dose will not cause any cardiovascular effects.

17. **The answer is B.** (Miller, 4/e. pp 428–429.) In a result probably related to the effect of neostigmine on pseudocholinesterase, 1 mg/kg of succinylcholine given 5 min after administration of 5 mg of neostigmine was shown to prolong its effect by 11 to 35 min.

18. **The answer is E.** (Miller, 4/e. pp 453–454.) Rocuronium is a steroidal nondepolarizing neuromuscular blocker that is an analog of vecuronium. Its onset of action is faster than that of vecuronium, with intubation conditions occurring in 60 to 90 s. Rocuronium may be an attractive alternative to succinylcholine for rapid control of the airway. It is of intermediate duration. Rocuronium is highly cardiac stable because it has only a mild vagolytic effect and does not cause histamine release. Breakdown occurs via hepatic (80 percent) and renal (20 percent) pathways, and there are no active metabolites of rocuronium.

19. **The answer is B (1, 3).** (Miller, 4/e. 304–307.) All opioids will block the sympathetic nervous system to a certain degree and also enhance parasympathetic and vagal tone. This effect tends to occur with large bolus doses of narcotics. Types of patients who are most susceptible to hypotension are those who are dependent on a high intrinsic sympathetic tone to maintain left ventricular function and those who are on exogenous catecholamines. A temporizing measure to avert hypotension is to supply exogenous catecholamines or anticholinergics (atropine or pancuronium). Volume loading and slow infusion of opioids also attenuate the hypotensive response. Hypotension also may be caused by histamine release. This can be attenuated by pretreatment with both H_1 and H_2 blockers.

20. **The answer is A (1, 2, 3).** (Miller, 4/e. pp 303–314.) All the opioids, except meperidine, cause some form of bradycardia. Fentanyl is thought to stimulate vagal tone, while sufentanil and alfentanil may block sympathetic tone. Morphine is thought to have direct effects on the SA node and AV conduction. Calcium channels are not known to be affected, although patients on calcium channel blockers may be at high risk to develop bradycardia from opioids.

21. **The answer is A (1, 2, 3).** (Miller, 4/e. 314–318.) Opioids do not have an effect on hypoxic pulmonary vasoconstriction. They cause respiratory depression by the following mechanisms. The opioid μ receptors in the central nervous system (brainstem) will mediate a decrease in responsiveness of ventilation to increasing levels of CO_2. This is seen as a decrease in the slope of the ventilatory/CO_2 curve, a shift to the right in minute ventilation responses to CO_2, and an increase in the apneic threshold to CO_2. Opioids will also decrease hypoxic drive. All these effects are additive when opioids are given along with other respiratory depressants.

22. **The answer is D (4).** (Miller, 4/e. 321–323.) Opioid rigidity tends to affect the thoracoabdominal musculature (wooden chest syndrome) and can make ventilation very difficult. The rigidity is not due to any motor end plate or neuromuscular junction interaction. Alfentanil causes the highest incidence of rigidity. The exact mechanism for opioid-induced rigidity is unknown. Incidence of rigidity is dose-dependent but can occur even if small doses of opioids are given quickly. Muscle relaxants or other anesthetic agents will reverse rigidity.

23. The answer is E (all). (Miller, 4/e. pp 320–321, 699–700.) Opioids are an extremely useful adjunct in the anesthetic management of patients undergoing neurosurgical procedures. However, opioids will cause respiratory depression, shift the CO_2 response curve downward and to the right, ablate the CO_2 apneic threshold, and inhibit hypoxic drive. Combined, these events can cause a mixed respiratory and metabolic acidosis and thereby lead to increased vasodilatation, CBF, and ICP. Also, opioids can cause sedation, which can be confusing in a patient with a worsening neurologic status.

24. The answer is B (1, 3). (Miller, 4/e. pp 345–346.) Remifentanil has an extremely quick onset, similar to alfentanil. Remifentanil is metabolized by nonspecific plasma and tissue esterases; its half-life is 10 min. Because of its quick onset and offset, remifentanil has utility in the outpatient setting. However, because of its quick offset, patients will be prone to postoperative pain. A postoperative pain modality must be in use for outpatients who receive remifentanil, such as local anesthetic field or nerve blocks, other opioids, or NSAIDs. Remifentanil, like all other narcotics, can illicit nausea and vomiting.

25. The answer is B (1, 3). (Miller, 4/e. pp 350–352.) Naloxone is primarily a μ receptor antagonist and has a lesser predilection for κ and δ receptors. Naltrexone can antagonize the effects of opioids for up to 24 h, while naloxone's duration of action is up to 45 min.

26. The answer is D (4). (Miller, 4/e. pp 2105–2106.) Morphine's peak effect occurs 1 to 2 h after IM and 20 min after IV administration. Because of its long duration of action, it has the greatest respiratory depressant effect on the newborn of all narcotics.

27. The answer is E (all). (Miller, 4/e. pp 321–323.) Elderly patients are most susceptible to truncal skeletal muscle rigidity with opioid agonists. This rigidity is not a direct effect of the opioid agonist on muscle fibers, but pretreatment with muscle relaxants can decrease or prevent its occurrence.

28. The answer is B (1, 3). (Miller, 4/e. pp 330–331.) Morphine has been shown to inhibit the vomiting center in the medulla. Opioids stimulate the dopamine receptors.

29. The answer is E (all). (Miller, 4/e. pp 352–353.) The ability of narcotics to depress ventilation can be potentiated by monoamine oxidase inhibitors, tricyclic antidepressants, and amphetamines. This may be related to the ability of these drugs to interfere with metabolism of narcotics. Atropine has been shown to antagonize narcotic-induced analgesia.

30. The answer is A (1, 2, 3). (Barash, 3/e. pp 375–376.) The addition of an opioid narcotic or a muscle relaxant has been shown to decrease MAC, as has a nerve block in the region of surgery. Mild isovolumic anemia has no effect on MAC.

31. The answer is D (4). (Miller, 4/e. pp 135–143.) Enflurane increases the resting Pa_{CO_2} more than does isoflurane in spontaneously ventilated unstimulated patients. The inhibitory effect of inhaled agents on ventilatory response to hypoxia is present at 0.1 MAC or higher. The depressant effect of inhaled agents on CO_2 response is decreased but not completely eliminated with surgical stimulation.

32. **The answer is D (4).** (Miller, 4/e. pp 101–123.) An increase in ventilation affects the rate of anesthetic rise more with the least soluble agents and less with the more soluble agents, but an increase in cardiac output affects the soluble agent more than the insoluble agent. Ventilation-perfusion abnormalities affect the anesthetic rise of insoluble agents more than that of the soluble agents. The solubility of the agents in decreasing order is ether > halothane > enflurane > nitrous oxide > desflurane.

33. **The answer is C (2, 4).** (Miller, 4/e. pp 1135–1142.) MAC is defined as a concentration that is a percentage of 1 atmosphere; it is therefore independent of elevation. At high altitudes, where atmospheric pressure is lower, a higher concentration of an agent must be delivered to achieve the same clinical effect that would be obtained at sea level. MAC is maximal between 6 months and 2 years of age. The physical property of general anesthetics that best correlates with anesthetic potency (or MAC) is lipid solubility. At equilibrium, partial pressures of inhaled anesthetics are equal in alveoli, blood, and brain.

34. **The answer is A (1, 2, 3).** (Miller, 4/e. pp 1135–1142.) MAC is age-dependent; it peaks in infancy and gradually decreases with age. MAC is directly correlated with the lipid solubility of the drug in question. Combining inhalation drugs can reduce the toxic effects of each while maintaining adequate anesthesia; the MACs are additive. The order of MAC is methyoxyflurane > halothane > isoflurane > enflurane > nitrous oxide.

35. **The answer is B (1, 3).** (Miller, 4/e. pp 145–146, 139–140, 146–152.) All inhaled agents depress baroreceptor function; isoflurane has the least depressant effect. All inhaled agents also decrease the slope of the ventilatory response curve to CO_2. This effect may cause postoperative respiratory compromise.

36. **The answer is E (all).** (Miller, 4/e. pp 120, 124–126.) Depression of ventilation is thought to be mediated by chemoreceptors in the medulla. The ventilatory response to hypoxia is mediated by peripheral chemoreceptors. A hypoxic patient will have a reduced drive to breathe. This has strong implications for the postanesthetic period. Isoflurane has little effect on cardiac output. Enflurane also decreases systemic vascular resistance, which is unchanged by halothane. In descending order of potency, enflurane, halothane, isoflurane, and nitrous oxide reduce the peak developed force and the rate of rise of developed force of myocardial muscle. The mechanism involves some aspect(s) of calcium physiology of the muscle cell.

37. The answer is D (4). (Miller, 4/e. pp 702–708.) Halothane increases cerebral blood flow the most, followed by enflurane and then isoflurane. Normally, changes in metabolic need and cerebral blood flow are in parallel. Inhaled agents cause an upcoupling of flow and metabolism; that is, they reduce cerebral metabolism while increasing cerebral blood flow. Isoflurane produces the smallest increase in cerebral blood flow and the greatest reduction in metabolic rate for oxygen, and in this respect it is the ideal inhaled anesthetic for the brain. Isoflurane is the least metabolized (0.2 percent), followed by enflurane (2 percent) and then halothane (20 percent).

38. The answer is C (2, 4). (Miller, 4/e. pp 101–123.) Essential to the second gas effect is that the first gas be delivered in high concentrations. It is the large volume of nitrous oxide that creates a vacuum in the alveoli so that more fresh gas is drawn in, thereby speeding uptake of the second gas. Insoluble agents, even in the absence of a high minute ventilation, achieve a rapid rate of rise of alveolar concentration. Soluble agents benefit the most from a high minute ventilation, which counteracts the effect of washout of anesthetic agent into the circulation. A blood gas partition coefficient of 2.4 means that the concentration of halothane in blood will be 2.4 times that in the gas phase but the partial pressures in blood and gas will be identical, which indicates that equilibrium has been achieved. The rate of rise of alveolar concentration with time is proportionate to solubility; i.e., the higher the solubility, the slower the rate of rise. From top to bottom, the curves in the diagram represent the rates of rise of nitrous oxide, desflurane, isoflurane, and halothane.

39. The answer is C (2, 4). (Miller, 4/e. pp 168–169, 172–173.) The fulminant form of halothane hepatitis is extremely rare in children, but it does occur. There is some evidence that enflurane hepatitis does occur. Isoflurane hepatitis has not been documented. The fulminant form is nearly uniformly fatal. It is now thought to be due to trifluoroacetic acid, an oxidative metabolite.

40. The answer is D (4). (Miller, 4/e. pp 1901–1902.) An increase in ADH secretion, potentiation of narcotics, and prolongation of nondepolarizing muscle relaxants are not known complications in patients who have undergone pneumoencephalography and then receive nitrous oxide. Pneumoencephalography is performed by the instillation of either air or oxygen into the subarachnoid space. Nitrous oxide can equilibrate with the gas-filled space and cause an increase in intracranial pressure, which leads to hypertension and bradycardia (Cushing's response). It is recommended that skull x-rays be obtained in patients who have undergone pneumoencephalography to discern if a gas bubble is still present preoperatively. It is also recommended that nitrous oxide not be used for 7 to 10 days after pneumoencephalography.

41. The answer is A (1, 2, 3). (Miller, 4/e. pp 162–163.) Hematopoietic and neurologic systems are both affected by prolonged nitrous oxide exposure. Nitrous oxide interacts with vitamin B_{12} to inactivate methionine synthetase. Methionine synthetase is essential in catalyzing the synthesis of methionine. Clinical syndromes of megaloblastic anemia and spinal cord degeneration result from nitrous oxide toxicity. Pretreatment with large doses of folinic acid can prevent bone marrow toxicity.

42. **The answer is B (1, 3).** (Miller, 4/e. pp 162–163, 178, 112–113, 105–106.) Significant volumes of N_2O can move into closed gas spaces. When these spaces contain gases less soluble than N_2O, such as nitrogen, N_2O diffuses into the space while nitrogen does not diffuse out. This results in either expansion or increase in the pressure of the space (depending on the compliance of the walls surrounding the space). N_2O oxidizes the cobalt in vitamin B_{12}, which inactivates methionine synthetase. Extreme consequences of this are megaloblastic hematopoiesis (after many hours of N_2O exposure). N_2O is not mutagenic. Teratogenicity by N_2O occurs in laboratory animals but has never been shown in humans. N_2O is 34 times more soluble than nitrogen in blood. When N_2O is discontinued, it rapidly enters alveoli and dilutes the gases, including oxygen, that are there.

43. **The answer is C (2, 4).** (Miller, 4/e. pp 991–992.) Patients on MAO inhibitors may have hemodynamic instability intraoperatively and are at risk to develop hyperpyrexic complications when narcotics, in particular meperidine, are given. These patients, however, are usually severely depressed, and so the discontinuation of these medications may be life-threatening. Careful monitoring and avoidance of certain drugs can allow successful anesthetic management of these patients without the discontinuation of MAO inhibitors. Direct α and β agonists should be titrated carefully because of possible denervation hypersensitivity.

44. **The answer is E (all).** (Miller, 4/e. pp 169–172.) Major metabolites of methoxyflurane include F^-, dichloroacetic acid. Enflurane, isoflurane, and desflurane, in decreasing order, produce F^- as a metabolite. F^- is a metabolite of the reductive pathway, not the oxidative metabolic pathway, for halothane.

45. **The answer is D (4).** (Miller, 4/e. pp 169–172.) Although all these agents produce F^- as a metabolite, only methoxyflurane has been shown to produce enough F^- to be nephrotoxic. Methoxyflurane nephrotoxicity is dose-dependent. There is much individual variation in the susceptibility of a patient to nephrotoxicity. However, because of the potential side effects, methoxyflurane is no longer in general clinical use.

46. **The answer is E (all).** (Miller, 4/e. 1026–1027.) Preoperative administration of clonidine in a single oral dose (4 to 5 μg/kg) will provide all these beneficial effects. In addition, this dose can diminish preoperative anxiety and lead to an awake but calm patient. Postoperatively, patients may require less narcotic for pain relief. There is no rebound hypertension effect after one oral dose. Rebound tends to occur only after 6 to 7 days of therapy.

47. The answer is C (2, 4). (Miller, 4/e. 1485–1486.) The first sign of nitroprusside toxicity is usually tachyphylaxis. Venous blood is often described as cherry red because of the abnormally high P_{O_2} that results when cyanide poisons the electron transport chain and renders tissues unable to utilize oxygen. Metabolic acidosis results. Nitroprusside is more effective than is nitroglycerin in lowering blood pressure but is much more toxic.

48. The answer is D (4). (Stoelting, *Pharmacology*, 2/e. pp 286, 441–442, 467, 472.) Digoxin inhibits the myocardial cell sodium-potassium pump, increasing intracellular calcium and improving contractility. Warfarin (Coumadin) interferes with the action (namely, carboxylation) of vitamin K in the synthesis of the listed factors. Antithrombin III, rather than thromboplastin, binds to heparin and results in inactivation of coagulation. Oral hypoglycemics improve tissue responsiveness to the effects of insulin as well as stimulating the release of insulin.

49. The answer is E (all). (Miller, 4/e. pp 990–993.) Phenothiazines block dopaminergic pathways, as do butyrophenones. They also produce sedation and depression. Of these three calcium channel blockers, verapamil is the greatest negative inotrope and the most effective for lowering heart rate, and nifedipine is the most effective for lowering blood pressure. A halothane-theophylline combination can be particularly deleterious, resulting in malignant dysrhythmias. Tricyclics also depress cardiac conduction.

50. The answer is A (1, 2, 3). (Miller, 4/e. p 2358.) Stellate ganglion block with bupivicaine will last for about 10 h. Intravenous preparations of guanethidine are not available in this country.

51. The answer is E (all). (Miller, 4/e. p 561.) The use of nonselective antagonists can induce bronchospasm as a result of the antagonism of $beta_2$ receptors in the airways that normally maintain bronchodilation. The decreased inotropy in patients whose cardiac function is marginal can cause cardiac failure. The effect of beta antagonism can mask the symptoms and signs of hypoglycemia. When used with calcium channel blockers, beta antagonists may prolong AV conduction and cause heart block.

52. The answer is C (2, 4). (Cousins, 2/e. pp 52, 114, 117.) Lipophilia is more important than pKa because this characteristic causes a large amount of the local anesthetic to be absorbed into surrounding neural tissues and remain in the area. A high degree of protein binding also causes a long duration of action. The diffusibility of a drug diminishes as ionization increases (it is the un-ionized form that is lipid-soluble and crosses membranes). The higher the pKa is, the less un-ionized form is present. Thus, agents with low pKa's (lidocaine, mepivacaine) have a faster onset of action, while tetracaine, with a high pKa, has a slow onset. Chloroprocaine is an exception; its pKa is high, and its onset of action is short. This may be due to the relatively high concentrations in which it is used. Vasoconstrictors increase depth and duration of blockade but decrease onset of block and peak plasma concentrations of local anesthetics.

53. **The answer is B (1, 3).** (Stoelting, *Pharmacology,* 2/e. pp 426–428.) The increased capacitance results in venous pooling and decreased heart size and wall tension. Total coronary blood flow is not increased in these patients. Uterine, ureteral, and smooth muscle tone in the biliary tract is decreased, along with esophageal muscle tone. Platelet aggregation is not affected; increased bleeding time is thought to be due to an increase in the size of the vessels.

54. **The answer is B (1, 3).** (Miller, 4/e. p 503.) Mixtures of two local anesthetics have not been demonstrated to have improvement in onset or duration over either drug alone. Nor have such mixtures been shown to reduce toxicity.

55. **The answer is B (1, 3).** (Miller, 4/e. pp 515–516.) Prilocaine causes methemoglobinemia. Na bisulfite was previously included in local anesthetic solutions and has been implicated in causing neurotoxicity.

56. **The answer is E (all).** (Miller, 4/e. p 502.) All these statements are true. The usual dose is 5 μg/mL. Although other vasoconstrictors have been tried, none is superior to epinephrine.

57. **The answer is E (all).** (Cousins, 2/e. pp 125, 137, 138.) Bupivacaine is more cardiotoxic than lidocaine, and signs of central nervous system toxicity while one is using the former agent should immediately prompt preparation for cardiotoxic effects. Etidocaine is a suitable agent only when profound muscle relaxation is required. Methemoglobinemia with prilocaine is often short-lived and self-limited but can be reversed with methylene blue 1 mg/kg. Although tetracaine is more toxic than lidocaine, its toxicity is dose-dependent, and both agents can be used safely to provide topical anesthesia.

58. **The answer is D (4).** (Miller, 4/e. p 502.) Epinephrine prolongs blockade of all local anesthetics when they are used for infiltration or peripheral nerve blocks because it delays intravascular absorption. Its effect is variable in epidural anesthesia. Prilocaine is not affected, probably because it is less of a vasodilator than are the others. Bupivacaine and etidocaine are highly lipophilic. They are quickly taken up and slowly released by adipose tissue in the epidural space, and so their duration of action is long; this effect is not enhanced by epinephrine. Phenylephrine is as effective as epinephrine in prolonging the duration of action of spinal blockade when given in equipotent doses.

59. **The answer is A (1, 2, 3).** (Miller, 4/e. pp 510–511.) Continuous infusion of bupivacaine in neonates needs to have a slower rate because these patients may have prolonged elimination of the drug because of immaturity of the metabolizing liver enzymes.

60. **The answer is B (1, 3).** (Miller, 4/e. pp 510–511.) Respiratory acidosis (elevation in Pa_{CO_2}) increases cerebral blood flow and enhances drug delivery. In addition, it lowers seizure threshold. The lowering of arterial pH decreases protein binding and thereby increases the proportion of free drug available for diffusion into the brain. Lowering of pH, however, increases the cationic form of local anesthetics and decreases the rate of diffusion through lipid barriers.

61. The answer is E (all). (Miller, 4/e. pp 511–512.) The primary cardiac effect of local anesthetics is that they decrease the maximum rate of depolarization in Purkinje fibers and ventricular muscle. This probably occurs through interference with fast sodium channels in cardiac membranes.

62. The answer is A (1, 2, 3). (Miller, 4/e. pp 512–515.) The negative inotropic effects of acidosis and hypoxia potentiate those of bupivacaine. Because bupivacaine blocks both slow calcium channels and fast sodium channels, reentrant rhythms similar to torsade de pointes can be seen with toxic doses. Studies comparing the greater cardiovascular toxicity of bupivacaine with that of lidocaine show higher concentrations of bupivacaine in myocardial tissue. Prilocaine, but not bupivacaine, is known to cause formation of methemoglobin, which can be reversed with methylene blue.

63. The answer is B (1, 3). (Miller, 4/e. pp 514–515.) Ropivacaine was developed because of the severe cardiac depression noted with bupivacaine overdose. It is slightly less potent in humans than bupivacaine, with a shorter duration of action. It also is cleared more rapidly from the peripheral circulation when given intravenously.

64. The answer is D (4). (Cousins, 2/e. pp 84–85.) Tetracaine, an ester local anesthetic, is metabolized by serum cholinesterase, as is succinylcholine. The other three are all amide drugs and undergo enzymatic degradation in the liver. Because ester hydrolysis occurs rapidly in serum, toxic effects of ester local anesthetics are short-lived. However, if the patient has the atypical enzyme, toxic effects may be prolonged.

65. The answer is C (2, 4). (Miller, 3/e. pp 489–491, 501.) The potency of a local anesthetic cannot be predicted on the basis of its amide or ester linkage. Removal of the linkage, however, decreases local anesthetic activity, and so there is an effect on potency. Addition of alkyl groups to either the aromatic or the amine end of the compound increases the hydrophobic nature and makes the local anesthetic more potent. Isolated nerve preparations often show major differences in drug potencies which do not hold clinically.

66. The answer is C (2, 4). (Cousins, 2/e. pp 113–114.) The onset of blockade depends primarily on the pKa of the drug. The closer the pKa is to physiologic pH, the faster the onset of block is because most of the drug will be non-ionized and will cross lipid membranes quickly. Chloroprocaine, with a pKa of 9.1, is an exception in that its onset of action is rapid despite a high pKa. A high concentration of drug (e.g., 2 to 3%) means that more molecules are available for penetration of nerves, and this factor outweighs the effect of the high pKa. Lipid solubility and potency have no effect on onset time.

67. The answer is D (4). (Cousins, 2/e. pp 114–115.) The pKa, the rate of onset, and whether the drug is an amide or an ester have little influence on the duration of action of local anesthetics. Protein binding is the major determinant of duration. However, vasodilating properties of the local anesthetics can influence duration. Local absorption of drugs terminates activity at the site of injection. Vasodilation precipitates absorption.

68. **The answer is D (4).** (Miller, 4/e. p 503.) By increasing the pH of some local anesthetics with bicarbonate, more drug will be in the un-ionized basic form and will cross membrane barriers more readily, hastening onset of the block. There is no effect on the depth of sensory or motor blockade or the duration of the block.

69. **The answer is D (4).** (Miller, 4/e. pp 503–504.) The dose of all local anesthetics needs to be reduced during pregnancy because sensitivity to these drugs may be increased. This occurs as early as the first trimester and may be more than just an anatomic consideration. Hormonal changes during pregnancy also may play a role.

70. **The answer is E (all).** (Stoelting, *Pharmacology,* 2/e. pp 102–110.) Hepatic clearance of methohexital is much higher than that of thiopental. Methohexital is approximately 2.5 times more potent than thiopental. Methohexital has produced seizure activity in patients undergoing resection of seizure-producing areas.

71. **The answer is E (all).** (Stoelting, *Pharmacology,* 2/e. pp 351–352.) Droperidol is an antagonist at the dopaminergic receptor. It is also a weak antagonist of peripheral alpha-adrenergic receptors. In patients with pheochromocytoma, extreme hypertension may result from droperidol, which releases catecholamines from the adrenal medulla as well as inhibiting the reuptake of catecholamines. Droperidol has no demonstrable effect on resting ventilation and CO_2 responsiveness.

72. **The answer is B (1, 3).** (Stoelting, *Pharmacology,* 2/e. pp 368–371.) Droperidol's antagonist properties are due to its effect on dopaminergic receptors; however, it is not effective against motion sickness. Resting ventilation is not altered by droperidol.

73. **The answer is A (1, 2, 3).** (Miller, 4/e. p 262.) Even though ketamine has minimal effects on central respiratory drive, when it is added to other respiratory depressants, there is an overall decrease in minute ventilation and even apnea. Ketamine may relax bronchial smooth muscle via two mechanisms: First, inhibition of reuptake of norepinephrine will stimulate bronchial $beta_2$ receptors; second, ketamine may directly relax bronchial smooth muscle. The net result is an improvement in pulmonary compliance. Even though ketamine maintains upper airway reflexes, silent aspiration has been known to occur. Ketamine causes hypersalivation, and an antisialagogue may be useful.

74. **The answer is B (1, 3).** (Stoelting, *Pharmacology,* 2/e. pp 134–141.) Ketamine is a phencyclidine derivative that produces a "dissociative anesthesia." It is metabolized extensively by the hepatic microsomal enzymes, but use of halothane or diazepam slows metabolism and prolongs the drug effects. Ketamine has excellent analgesic properties.

75. The answer is A (1, 2, 3). (Miller, 4/e. p 268.) Porphyria is not triggered by etomidate. Nausea and vomiting are associated with etomidate, much to the distress of patients. There is adrenal suppression of cortisol release, but it is unclear whether this is clinically significant.

76. The answer is A (1, 2, 3). (Miller, 4/e. pp 266–268.) Etomidate does not alter hepatic function. It has the desirable properties of maintaining hemodynamic stability, cerebral protection, and respiratory function.

77. The answer is B (1, 3). (Miller, 4/e. p 266.) Etomidate does not alter brainstem evoked potentials. It is epileptogenic and has been used to identify seizure foci for removal. Etomidate maintains cerebral autoregulation and causes decreases in ICP, CBF, and $CMRO_2$, resulting in a net increase in CPP. This maintains a favorable balance of cerebral oxygen supply and demand.

78. The answer is A (1, 2, 3). (Miller, 4/e. pp 269–270.) Propofol is a 2,6 substituted phenol (2,6-diisopropylphenol) with hypnotic properties. It is highly lipid-soluble and is now prepared with soybean oil. Propofol is rapidly metabolized and cleared by the liver. It is metabolized so rapidly that it is believed that another organ, such as the lung, may contribute to its metabolism.

79. The answer is A (1, 2, 3). (Miller, 4/e. p 272.) Propofol leads to decreases in blood pressure, cardiac output, and cardiac index. It decreases venous return to the right heart via venodilation. Propofol also decreases myocardial contractility and afterload. There is no reflex increase in heart rate in response to the decreased stroke volume because baroreceptors are reset rather than inhibited. Propofol does not sensitize the myocardium to dysrhythmias.

80. The answer is D (4). (Miller, 4/e. pp 270–271.) Propofol is neither an antianalgesic nor an analgesic. Patients tend to awaken from propofol with a sense of well-being and sometimes even euphoria. Stays in the recovery room after use of propofol are shorter, because of its shorter half-life, than those after barbiturates. Propofol causes decreases in ICP and IOP. Propofol affects the respiratory and cardiovascular systems in a fashion similar to that of barbiturates. Cardiovascular depression had been reported to be somewhat greater with propofol use.

81. The answer is D (4). (Miller, 4/e. p 272.) Propofol does not potentiate neuromuscular blockade or suppress adrenal function. Neither is it a known trigger of MH. It does have antiemetic properties and has been used to treat postoperative nausea.

82. The answer is C (2, 4). (Miller, 4/e. p 270.) Women have a larger volume of distribution and an increased clearance but comparable elimination half-life for propofol compared with men. Hepatic diseases decrease its clearance, while renal diseases have no significant effect.

83. **The answer is A (1, 2, 3).** (Miller, 4/e. p 231.) GABA receptor activity of thiopental correlates well with its potency. Thiopental is quickly delivered to highly perfused organs such as the brain but is also rapidly transferred away. Though these is a high affinity of thiopental for fat tissue, these cells are poorly perfused and thus do not receive much drug in the usual clinical setting.

84. **The answer is D (4).** (Miller, 4/e. pp 236–241.) The main effect of thiopental and methohexital is venodilation. Heart rate is increased; systemic vascular resistance does not decrease. Intraarterial thiopental at high injection rates with large volumes and at solution strengths $> 25\%$ can result in endarteritis and severe pain and, in extreme cases, gangrene and tissue necrosis. With initial administration of thiopental, slowing of brain waves occurs with progression to delta and theta activity, followed by burst suppression and electrical silence. Barbiturates induce δ-aminolevulinic acid synthetase in the liver, which stimulates porphyria biosynthesis. No special precautions need be taken with porphyria cutanea tarda.

85. **The answer is B (1, 3).** (Miller, 4/e. pp 237–238.) Barbiturates have a central respiratory depressant effect that includes a decrease in the rate and depth of breathing and a decreased response to hypercarbia and hypoxemia. Unlike ketamine, barbiturates do not cause bronchodilation or significant salivation. Thiopental has been reported to trigger bronchospasm, but this is most likely due to manipulation of the airway in a very lightly anesthetized patient.

86. **The answer is A (1, 2, 3).** (Miller, 4/e. pp 236–237.) Barbiturates do not alter somatosensory evoked potentials even after they evoke burst suppression (isoelectric flat line) EEG. In a dose-dependent fashion, barbiturates slow the EEG pattern from the awake alpha phase straight through to burst suppression and flat EEG. Barbiturates decrease $CMRO_2$, CBF, and ICP but maintain CPP because ICP is decreased more than is mean arterial blood pressure. They significantly reduce IOP.

87. **The answer is C (2, 4).** (Miller, 4/e. p 238.) Barbiturates do not have any direct or indirect effect on sensitization of the heart to dysrhythmias. They directly decrease sympathetic outflow from the central nervous system. In addition, barbiturates cause venous pooling, which decreases blood return to the right heart and decreases myocardial contractility. This will cause a decreased cardiac output. In response to these changes, via baroreceptor reflexes, heart rate will increase, and this will offset somewhat the decrease in cardiac output. The net result, even with the compensatory increase in heart rate, is a decrease in cardiac output.

88. The answer is E (all). (Miller, 4/e. pp. 249, 254–255.) The elimination half-life of midazolam is 1.7 to 2.6 h, while that for diazepam is 20 to 50 h. The reduction in systemic vascular resistance by midazolam results in a slight decrease in blood pressure. The mechanism for the synergistic hemodynamic effects of benzodiazepines and opioids is unknown but may be related to decreased sympathetic tone. Hemodynamic effects with midazolam are minimal, and there is no venoirritant effect. Respiratory depression is dose-related and is more severe in patients with chronic obstructive pulmonary disease (COPD); it can progress to apnea.

89. The answer is A (1, 2, 3). (Miller, 4/e. pp 256–257.) Flumazenil is the first antagonist of benzodiazepines (midazolam, diazepam, and lorazepam) to be used clinically. It competes with benzodazepines for benzodiazepine receptor sites and has little activity once it binds to receptor sites. Flumazenil reverses the unconsciousness, respiratory depression, sedation, and amnesia caused by benzodiazepines. It does have weak intrinsic agonist effects. When flumazenil is used to reverse the unwanted side effects of benzodiazepine, there is no sympathetic nervous system stimulation unless the patient is physically dependent on benzodiazepine.

90. The answer is E (all). (Miller, 4/e. p 250.) Advanced age reduces the clearance of diazepam and midazolam but not that of lorazepam. Obesity does not alter the clearance of benzodiazepines, and so an infusion should be based on lean body weight. However, because the drugs are stored in fat, an induction dose needs to be increased.

91. The answer is A (1, 2, 3). (Miller, 4/e. pp 426–428.) Succinylcholine is safe in cerebral palsy, but hyperkalemia can occur in the conditions listed. Myalgias are effectively prevented by pretreatment with nondepolarizing muscle relaxants. Stimulation of muscarinic receptors increases the risk of bradydysrhythmias. Intraocular pressure cannot be reliably prevented with pretreatment.

92. The answer is A (1, 2, 3). (Miller, 4/e. pp 424–425.) Pseudocholinesterase levels may be reduced in pregnancy as a result of increased plasma volume. Production may be decreased in the presence of liver disease or cytotoxic drugs. Patients with a dibucaine number of 20 have atypical pseudocholinesterase, but the level is not reduced.

93. The answer is A (1, 2, 3). (Miller, 4/e. p 441.) Atracurium, curare, and metocurine all cause release of histamine in vivo. With rapid injection, this may be associated with significant hypotension. Vecuronium does not cause release of histamine.

94. The answer is A (1, 2, 3). (Miller, 4/e. pp 472–473.) Burn injury causes a marked increase in nicotinic acetylcholine receptors over the entire muscle surface, which leads to a hyperkalemic response to SCh within a few days of a burn and a relative resistance to nondepolarizing relaxants. The hyperkalemic response to SCh depends on the dose of SCh but not on the extent of the burn. The susceptibility to this hyperkalemic response persists as long as infection is present and healing is still going on.

95. **The answer is A (1, 2, 3).** (Miller, 4/e. pp 427, 473.) Hyperkalemia is a contraindication for the use of SCh. Patients with hemiplegia may have an exaggerated release of potassium after receiving SCh. The magnitude of the hyperkalemic response does not correlate closely with the magnitude of burn injury, and so any significant burn warrants conservative treatment. Patients with hemiplegia may have an exaggerated release of potassium after receiving SCh, which may lead to dysrhythmias. Cerebral palsy is not a contraindication to the use of succinylcholine.

96. **The answer is C (2, 4).** (Miller, 4/e. pp 424, 429–430.) Hydrolysis by pseudocholinesterase limits the duration of action of succinylcholine by rapidly depleting the amount of drug that reaches the motor end plate. However, termination of drug effect is due to diffusion of succinylcholine away from the end plate. Eighty percent inhibition suggests normal pseudocholinesterase. Homozygous abnormal enzyme is only 20 percent inhibited by dibucaine; such patients typically have a dibucaine number of approximately 20. Train-of-four stimulation will show transition from a phase I to a phase II block. If succinylcholine is stopped at this point, normal neuromuscular function will return rapidly. Neostigmine most effectively inhibits acetylcholinesterase, but it also partially inhibits pseudocholinesterase and therefore can prolong a succinylcholine-induced block.

97. **The answer is E (all).** (Miller, 4/e. pp 429–465.) Neostigmine and pyridostigmine are cholinesterase inhibitors. As such, they inhibit pseudocholinesterase, the enzyme that metabolizes SCh. This accounts for the prolongation of effect of SCh when it is given after administration of neostigmine and pyridostigmine. Magnesium has been shown to enhance the effect of both nondepolarizing muscle relaxants and SCh, as has quinidine, which has prejunctional effects on muscle membranes.

98. **The answer is C (2, 4).** (Rogers, p 2588. Miller, 4/e. pp 463–465. Rogers, p. 232.) $Pa_{CO_2} > 50$ torr can cause failure to reverse a nondepolarizing block. Metabolic alkalosis, but not acidosis, will prevent antagonism of a nondepolarizing block. The reason for this is unknown. The mechanisms for antibiotic-induced augmentation are varied, and the response to antagonism by neostigmine in this setting is unpredictable. Magnesium decreases the amount of acetylcholine released from nerve terminals, the excitability of the muscle cell, and the end-plate potential. Quinidine appears to act on the prejunctional membrane.

99. **The answer is B (1, 3).** (Miller, 4/e. pp 463–465.) Infants have an increased sensitivity to vecuronium, which also has a longer duration of action in infants. Hypothermia markedly prolongs the neuromuscular blockade of atracurium. Although volume of distribution is increased for atracurium in neonates and infants, the duration of action remains unchanged because of the increase in clearance in younger patients. Renal failure delays clearance of acetylcholinesterase inhibitors to the same extent as that of muscle relaxants; therefore, no adjustment for dosing of acetylcholinesterase inhibitors is needed.

100. The answer is A (1, 2, 3). (Miller, 4/e. pp 463–464.) Antibiotics, except for penicillins and cephalosporins, prolong the action of nondepolarizing muscle relaxants. Local anesthetics and furosemide also have been shown to prolong this action. In contrast, phenytoin apparently causes resistance to nondepolarizing muscle relaxants.

101. The answer is A (1, 2, 3). (Miller, 4/e. pp 449, 451–452, 468, 474.) Tachycardia induced by pancuronium is secondary to its inhibition of catecholamine reuptake, ganglionic stimulation, and vagolytic effects. A *d*-tubocurarine neuromuscular block is markedly augmented by inhaled anesthetics, more so than vecuronium or rocuronium. Laudanosine's CNS stimulatory effects have not been shown to have serious clinical consequences. Atracurium is not contraindicated in patients with epilepsy.

102. The answer is B (1, 3). (Miller, 4/e. pp 418, 427.) Metocurine and gallamine are entirely dependent on renal excretion, and their duration of action is prolonged in renal failure patients. Vecuronium is much less dependent on the kidney for elimination, and its duration of action is not prolonged in renal failure. Atracurium pharmacokinetics are unaffected in cirrhosis.

103. The answer is D (4). (Miller, 4/e. pp 461–463.) The augmentation effect is dose-dependent for all agents. Only enflurane has been shown to augment muscle relaxants in a time-dependent fashion. No demonstrable effect at the cholinergic receptors has been shown.

104. The answer is E (all). (Miller, 4/e. pp 746–748.) Extrajunctional receptors are under the trophic influence of neural modulation; i.e., denervation makes them atrophy. Therefore, before full maturation of the neuromuscular junction prior to age 2, both junctional and extrajunctional receptors are made. In addition, they are made when neuronal activity is impaired or absent.

105. The answer is D (4). (Miller, 4/e. p 751.) Neostigmine, edrophonium, and pyridostigmine all contain quaternary ammonium ions and do not penetrate the blood-brain barrier; therefore, they exert no effect in the CNS.

106. The answer is D (4). (Miller, 4/e. pp 750–751, 567.) Organophosphates, not edrophonium, produce irreversible inhibition of acetylcholinesterase. Physostigmine and neostigmine work by forming carbamyl esters with acetylcholinesterase. Edrophonium has a faster onset of action than do neostigmine and pyridostigmine and is eliminated primarily via the kidneys.

107. The answer is B (1, 3). (Stoelting, *Pharmacology,* 2/e. pp 243–244.) Glycopyrrolate is a poorly soluble quaternary ammonium compound. Secondary to its poor lipid solubility, it does not cross membranes easily. It is a less potent antisialagogue than scopolamine but is more potent than atropine. Glycopyrrolate has minimal effects on pupillary size.

108. **The answer is A (1, 2, 3).** (Miller, 4/e. pp 739–740, 748.) Larger than normal doses of muscle relaxants are required to cause relaxation in patients with extrajunctional receptors. The difference in duration of action between succinylcholine and acetylcholine is due mainly to the proximity of the enzyme to its respective target molecule. Acetylcholinesterase is present right at the acetylcholine receptor, and the metabolism of acetylcholine occurs instantaneously as acetylcholine is released. Succinylcholine must diffuse out of the synaptic cleft into the bloodstream before it reaches its enzyme.

109. **The answer is C (2, 4).** (Miller, 4/e. pp 737–740.) Calcium channel blockers have little effect on the release of acetylcholine. When acetylcholine reacts with the nicotinic acetylcholine receptor, the net electrical effect is depolarization, which initiates an end-plate potential and results in muscle contraction. Acetylcholinesterase resides in the synaptic cleft, where acetylcholine is broken down. There is one beta, one delta, and one epsilon subunit as well as the alpha subunits on the acetylcholine receptor.

110. **The answer is B (1, 3).** (Stoelting, *Pharmacology,* 2/e. p 232. Rogers, p 1501.) Miosis, bronchoconstriction, increased bladder and decreased sphincter tone, increased salivation, slowing at the sinus node, and increased gastrointestinal tone are all results of muscarinic stimulation. Stimulation of autonomic ganglia occurs via nicotinic receptors.

111. **The answer is A (1, 2, 3).** (Miller, 4/e. p 441.) Vecuronium and pancuronium are classified as steroids, while *d*-tubocurarine, metocurine, and atracurium are classified as benzylisoquinolines. Neuromuscular blockers from the same class are additive when used in combination, while those from different classes behave in a synergistic manner.

112. **The answer is E (all).** (Miller, 4/e. pp 420, 1352.) Respiratory acidosis, due to hypoventilation, may develop after head lift or sustained tetanus has been achieved, and this will potentiate any residual neuromuscular blockade. Thus, patients who have been given muscle relaxants need a period of close observation even after "reversal" has been confirmed clinically or with a neuromuscular blockade monitor. With sustained tetanus at 100 Hz, 50 percent of receptors may still be blocked, whereas with a normal train-of-four, 75 percent may be blocked. The diaphragm may require up to twice as much muscle relaxant as do peripheral muscles to show similar blockade.

113. **The answer is D (4).** (Stoelting, *Pharmacology,* 2/e. pp 333–334. Kaplan, p. 968. Rogers, p 1488.) Muscarmic anticholinergic drugs are protective against brochospasm, as in the antiasthmatic drug ipratropium. Trimethaphan and other ganglionic blocking drugs affect both sympathetic and parasympathetic nervous systems to different degrees. Because of this, the systemic effects of these drugs are unpredictable. Ephedrine is not a catecholamine. Its predominant effects are indirect, e.g., release of norepinephrine. It also has direct stimulant effects on adrenergic receptors. The venoconstrictor effect is mediated by stimulation of alpha receptors on capacitance vessels, and norepinephrine is the most potent agent in this regard.

114. The answer is C (2, 4). (Miller, 4/e. pp 524, 528–529.) Preganglionic parasympathetic fibers synapse in the organ they innervate and are therefore long compared with sympathetic preganglionic fibers, which synapse close to the spinal cord in ganglia and then send out long postganglionic fibers to distant sites. The parasympathetic system also liberates acetylcholine from the preganglionic fibers, but in this case to muscarinic receptors. Several sympathetic levels innervate a single sensory dermatome. The celiac ganglion innervates the liver, pancreas, spleen, stomach, small colon, proximal large colon, and kidneys.

115. The answer is B (1, 3). (Miller, 4/e. p 568.) Ganglionic blocking drugs, such as trimethaphan, have effects on both sympathetic and parasympathetic receptors. Sympathetic blockade results in mydriasis, vasodilation, decreased cardiac output, and decreased venous return, which leads to hypotension. Parasympathetic blockade leads to tachycardia.

116. The answer is B (1, 3). (Miller, 4/e. pp 558–559, 561.) Metoprolol, atenolol, esmolol, betaxolol, and bevantolol are beta$_1$ selective drugs. The short half-life of esmolol is due to its rapid hydrolysis by esterases. As most of these drugs undergo hepatic metabolism, there is a significant first-pass hepatic extraction, which lowers serum levels compared with those of parenterally administered drug. Only nadolol and atenolol are predominantly excreted by the kidney.

117. The answer is A (1, 2, 3). (Miller, 4/e. pp 545–546.) Beta receptor density can be changed by a number of physiologic and pharmacologic influences. Chronic stimulation by agonists, hypothyroidism, and corticosteroids decrease receptor density and responsiveness. This is called *down-regulation.* Chronic administration of antagonists and hyperthyroidism increase receptor density and responsiveness. This called *up-regulation.* Diabetes mellitus is not known to affect beta receptor sensitivity.

118. The answer is A (1, 2, 3). (Miller, 4/e. pp 552–555.) Dopamine has direct and indirect receptor effects. It also has effects on specific dopaminergic receptors in the splanchnic and renal beds. Epinephrine has direct effects on both alpha and beta receptors. Ephedrine has both direct and indirect receptor effects. Release of norepinephrine from indirect stimulation causes both alpha and beta$_1$ effects.

119. The answer is C (2, 4). (Miller, 4/e. p 563.) ACE is located predominantly in lung endothelium, where it converts angiotensin I to angiotensin II. Angioedema can be caused by all ACE inhibitors and is especially common after the first dose. While calcium channel blockers or digoxin should be used very cautiously in patients on a beta blocker because of the risk of undesirable dysrhythmias, there is no such concern with the ACE inhibitor combination.

120. **The answer is C (2, 4).** (Miller, 4/e. p 561.) Hypoglycemia is not caused by beta blockers. Beta blockers may in fact reduce insulin output and result in hyperglycemia. Beta blockers should be used with caution in diabetic patients because they may mask signs of hypoglycemia, i.e., tachycardia and tremor. Beta antagonists may reduce hepatic clearance of lidocaine. Limetidone may increase plasma concentrations of some beta blockers by decreasing hepatic perfusion. There is no effect on laryngospasm, although bronchospasm may be triggered by beta blockade of beta$_2$-mediated bronchodilation.

121. **The answer is E (all).** (Miller, 4/e. pp 451–453.) Patients with hepatic failure also may have varying degrees of cardiac and renal compromise. *Cis*-atracurium may be a useful nondepolarizing relaxant in this population of patients for the following reasons: nondependence on hepatic and/or renal metabolism, i.e., Hoffmann elimination and ester hydrolysis, and a stable hemodynamic profile in that there is no histamine release.

122. **The answer is B (1, 3).** (Stoelting, *Pharmacology,* 3/e. pp 450–452.) Mannitol is a nonmetabolized six-carbon sugar. No filtered drug is reabsorbed from the renal tubules. Urea, not mannitol, is associated with venous thrombosis.

123. **The answer is C (2, 4).** (Stoelting, *Pharmacology,* 2/e. pp 357–362.) Caution is necessary when using local anesthetics in patients on verapamil. Nifedipine has a greater effect on vascular smooth muscles than does verapamil.

124. **The answer is A (1, 2, 3).** (Stoelting, *Pharmacology,* 2/e. pp 285–292.) Digoxin, as opposed to digitoxin, undergoes minimal metabolism. Dihydrodigoxin is the inactive metabolite formed from digoxin.

125. **The answer is C (2, 4).** (Stoelting, *Pharmacology,* 2/e. pp 293–294.) Amrinone is neither a catecholamine nor a glycoside but a bipyridine derivative that produces dose-dependent increases in cardiac output and decreases in LVEDP. Amrinone does not potentiate toxicity. Chronic use of amrinone may result in thrombocytopenia.

126. **The answer is A (1, 2, 3).** (Stoelting, *Pharmacology,* 2/e. pp 448–449.) The reabsorption of sodium and chloride ions is blocked in the medullary portion of the loop of Henle. Furosemide augments blockade by nondepolarizing muscle relaxants; theories to explain this involve hypokalemia and decreased acetylcholine release. The depletion of myocardial potassium by furosemide renders the heart more susceptible to digitalis toxicity. Renal clearance of lithium is decreased and plasma levels of lithium are increased when furosemide is given.

127. **The answer is B (1, 3).** (Stoelting, *Pharmacology,* 2/e. pp 313, 315, 319–321.) Guanethidine and captopril work only on peripheral receptors; both cause vasodilation. Alpha-methyldopa and clonidine have central alpha$_2$ activity. This central effect can cause sedation, and both agents are known to decrease general anesthetic requirements.

128. **The answer is C (2, 4).** (Miller, 4/e. p 563.) Captopril blocks the enzyme that converts angiotensin I to angiotensin II. It decreases plasma aldosterone with slight increases in plasma potassium levels. Renin levels are increased because of lack of inhibition from angiotensin II.

MACHINERY

Directions: Each item below contains four or five suggested responses. Select the **one best** response to each question.

129. The "fail-safe" system of an anesthesia machine

(A) prevents a hypoxic mixture if there is a leak in the system upstream from the vaporizers

(B) is placed between the flowmeters and the patients as an O_2 sensor to prevent a hypoxic mixture

(C) is a link between the flowmeters in modern machines to prevent a hypoxic mixture

(D) opens the O_2 tank supply to the anesthesia machine if the wall supply of O_2 fails

(E) senses a drop in main O_2 pressure and proportionately decreases N_2O supply to prevent a hypoxic mixture

130. In a volume-cycled ventilator,

(A) preset volume determines the end of the inspiratory phase

(B) preset time determines the beginning of the expiratory phase

(C) the volume of gas delivered to the patient is difficult to control

(D) pathophysiologic changes in the patient can affect the volume delivery

(E) variations in airway pressure waveforms are difficult to accomplish

131. N_2O and O_2 cylinders on the anesthesia machine should be turned off until needed because

(A) they bypass the fail-safe valve

(B) pin indexing is not used on these cylinders, which may lead to errors and hypoxic mixtures

(C) the flush valve will not work with the tanks

(D) the tanks are at a much higher pressure than the wall supply and will be preferentially and rapidly depleted

(E) silent emptying of the tanks will occur over time when machine pressure is lower than cylinder pressure

132. All the following statements concerning oxygen E cylinders are true EXCEPT

(A) as the tank empties, remaining gauge pressure is proportionate to the number of liters of oxygen left in the cylinder

(B) a full cylinder contains 625 L of oxygen

(C) a full cylinder has a pressure of 2000 PSIG

(D) the pressure-reducing valve on the cylinder will allow oxygen to exit at 45 to 50 PSIG

(E) the color of the cylinder is yellow

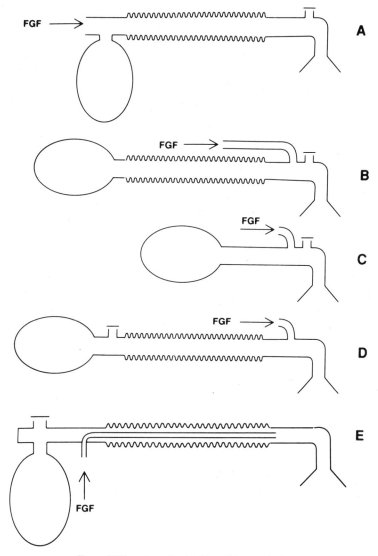

From Miller, *Anesthesia,* 3/e, with permission.

133. Which of the systems above is most efficient at preventing rebreathing when low fresh gas flow (FGF) is used during spontaneous ventilation?

134. Which of the circuits above can be dangerous because the fresh gas flow can be kinked or disconnected without detection, leading to hypercarbia and hypoxemia?

135. True statements concerning the nitrous oxide (N_2O) E cylinder include

    (A) the cylinder is red in color
    (B) N_2O is in the state of a compressed gas
    (C) there is approximately 1600 L of N_2O in an E cylinder
    (D) the relationship between decrease in pressure and amount of N_2O left is proportionate
    (E) a full N_2O E cylinder has 2000 PSIG

136. When a full E tank of oxygen is used to transport an intubated patient at a flow of 6 L/min, oxygen will run out in

    (A) 30 min
    (B) 55 min
    (C) 80 min
    (D) 110 min
    (E) 120 min

137. The designation "IT" on an endotracheal tube refers to

    (A) sterility test
    (B) tissue toxicity test
    (C) nonflammability
    (D) radio-opacity
    (E) allergic potential

138. The zero reference point of the system is the

    (A) transducer dome
    (B) right atrium
    (C) stopcock closest to the vessel cannulated
    (D) stopcock used in calibration
    (E) strain gauge head

139. In using transducers to monitor blood pressures,

    (A) air bubbles decrease dampening of the waveform
    (B) air bubbles decrease the elastic component of the system
    (C) tubing diameter is of little importance in the monitoring system
    (D) increased tubing length can cause excessive "ringing" in the system
    (E) excessive "ringing" in the system can be controlled by decreasing dampening

140. Which of the following is the most commonly employed noninvasive method of measuring blood pressure?

    (A) Doppler technique for detecting blood flow distal to the cuff
    (B) Ultrasonic technique for sensing the motion of the arterial wall
    (C) Detection of auscultatory frequency
    (D) Oscillometric technique

141. Which of the following has no effect on pulse oximetry?

    (A) Methylene blue
    (B) Methemoglobinemia
    (C) Bright ambient lights
    (D) Polycythemia

142. Five minutes after a single dose of 100 mg succinylcholine, the pattern in response to train-of-four peripheral nerve stimulation in a 70-kg man is most likely to be

    (A) 1 twitch
    (B) 2 twitches
    (C) 3 twitches
    (D) no twitch

Directions: Each question below contains four suggested responses of which **one or more** is correct. Select:

(A)	if	**1, 2, and 3**	are correct
(B)	if	**1 and 3**	are correct
(C)	if	**2 and 4**	are correct
(D)	if	**4**	is correct
(E)	if	**1, 2, 3, and 4**	are correct

143. Compared with low flow rates, high flow rates cause

(1) less rebreathing
(2) less predictability of the inspired anesthetic concentration
(3) a greater tendency toward atmospheric pollution
(4) a higher humidity in inspired gases

144. True statements about soda lime include

(1) the smaller the granules of soda lime, the more surface area there is for absorption of CO_2
(2) air flow resistance increases with smaller granules
(3) dye indicators added to soda lime change colors because of the change in pH of exhausted soda lime
(4) soda lime contains the water needed to catalyze the CO_2 absorption reaction

145. Automated blood pressure devices measure blood pressure by the oscillometric principle. With this method,

(1) systolic and diastolic pressures are measured and the mean is derived
(2) the systolic point is the pressure of maximum oscillation
(3) diastole is measured when pulse amplitude begins to decline
(4) mean pressure is measured and systolic and diastolic pressures are derived

146. Manual methods of blood pressure monitoring rely on Korotkoff sounds. Errors of measurement occur when

(1) stethoscope tubing is too long
(2) the manometer is improperly calibrated
(3) cardiogenic shock is present
(4) vasopressors are used

147. Use of the sphygmomanometer is accurately characterized by which of the following statements?

(1) Cuff width should be 40 to 50 percent of the circumference of the limb
(2) Narrow cuffs will lead to artificially low blood pressure readings
(3) Rapid cuff deflation will give the most accurate readings
(4) When severely artherosclerotic vessels underlie the cuff, artificially high blood pressure readings will be taken

148. Complications of automated blood pressure monitoring include

(1) nerve paresthesias
(2) compartment syndrome
(3) superficial thrombophlebitis
(4) limited perfusion to distal extremity

149. In which of the following clinical conditions will the thermal dilution technique of cardiac output measurement be INACCURATE?

(1) Infusion of a large volume of fluid into the right side of the heart
(2) Febrile patients
(3) The presence of a left-to-right shunt
(4) Patients with isolated right-sided cardiac failure

SUMMARY OF DIRECTIONS

A	B	C	D	E
1,2,3 only	1,3 only	2,4 only	4 only	All are correct

150. In measuring cardiac output with a thermodilution catheter, accuracy is increased by

    (1) multiple measurements
    (2) the use of iced injectate
    (3) measurements made in the same phase of the respiratory cycle
    (4) measurements made in conjunction with the QRS phase of the ECG

151. Important conditions for the use of the continuous mixed venous oxygen saturation catheter as a cardiac output monitor include the presence of constant

    (1) Pa_{O_2}
    (2) oxygen consumption
    (3) hemoglobin concentration
    (4) heart rate

152. Advantages offered by transesophageal echocardiography include

    (1) the use of a highly specific marker of severe myocardial ischemia
    (2) a stable, continuous monitor of cardiac function
    (3) objective evaluation of function
    (4) ability to accurately visualize abnormal anatomy of the heart

153. The risk of pulmonary artery rupture with PA catheters increases with

    (1) rapid inflation of balloon
    (2) peripheral migration of catheter
    (3) high inflation volumes
    (4) elderly patients

154. In transesophageal echocardiography, the basic *three-chamber view* shows the function of

    (1) aortic and mitral valves simultaneously
    (2) left ventricular outflow tract
    (3) left atrium
    (4) right ventricular outflow tract

155. Conditions that may prevent the pulmonary artery diastolic pressure from accurately reflecting LVEDV include

    (1) hypoxia
    (2) hyperthermia
    (3) hypercarbia
    (4) tachycardia

156. True statements about pulmonary arterial pressure monitoring of the normal heart include

    (1) phasic blood flow in the occluded pulmonary vessel is stopped when the balloon is properly wedged
    (2) the catheter tip must rest in zone II of the lung for accurate measurements
    (3) pulmonary artery occlusion pressure (PAOP) provides an accurate estimate of left heart preload
    (4) positive-end expiratory pressure (PEEP) has no effect on pulmonary artery diastolic pressure (PADP)

157. True statements regarding a left atrial pressure tracing include which of the following?

(1) The v wave corresponds to filling of the left atrium during ventricular disastole

(2) If a left atrial pressure tracing is superimposed on the electrocardiogram at the same instant in time, the v wave occurs simultaneously with the PR interval

(3) The c wave is simultaneous with mitral valve opening

(4) The a wave represents atrial systole

158. CVP monitoring reflects

(1) intravascular volume

(2) intrinsic vascular tone of thoracic vessels

(3) contractile function of the right heart

(4) driving force for filling the right heart

159. True statements regarding pulse oximeters include which of the following?

(1) They are more sensitive to changes in arterial oxygenation than are measurements of arterial blood gases (ABGs) at a P_{O_2} greater than 100

(2) They compare the relative absorbance of 4 wavelengths of light to determine fractional oxygen saturation

(3) They give a falsely low oxygen saturation in patients with elevated serum bilirubin

(4) They may give a falsely high oxygen saturation in patients with high carboxyhemoglobin concentrations secondary to smoke inhalation

160. The Allen test is correctly described by which of the following statements?

(1) Ischemic complications are far less likely to occur if the test is normal than if it is abnormal

(2) It is abnormal in patients who later develop ischemic complications from radial arterial cannulation

(3) A normal test correlates well with the presence of distal blood flow as assessed by injection of fluorescein dye

(4) The test can be used to assess ulnar arterial patency when cannulation of the radial artery is contemplated

161. True statements regarding capnography include

(1) the slope of the expiratory upstroke on the capnogram varies inversely with the duration of exhalation; i.e., the steeper the slope, the shorter the exhalation

(2) a large pulmonary embolus or severe bronchospasm will result in an elevated end-tidal CO_2

(3) the presence of CO_2 rebreathing can be detected by an elevated inspiratory baseline on the capnogram

(4) a capnometer uses ultraviolet light to measure CO_2 absorption

SUMMARY OF DIRECTIONS

A	B	C	D	E
1,2,3 only	1,3 only	2,4 only	4 only	All are correct

162. Which of the following conditions would be likely to result in an increased end-tidal CO_2 in the presence of constant controlled ventilation?

    (1) Pyrexia
    (2) Release of tourniquet
    (3) Administration of bicarbonate
    (4) Pulmonary embolus

163. Capnometry is accurately characterized by which of the following statements?

    (1) All the following can elevate end-tidal CO_2: alveolar hypoventilation, insufflation of CO_2 into the abdominal cavity, and bicarbonate therapy
    (2) Shunt (as in a pneumothorax) produces a widened gradient of arterial to end-tidal CO_2
    (3) During mechanical positive pressure ventilation, end-tidal CO_2 will decrease if fresh gas flow is increased from 5 to 10 L/min, even without changing the ventilatory settings on the ventilator
    (4) A potential problem in the use of capnometers is that an esophageal intubation can go undetected (i.e., a normal CO_2 tracing will appear on the capnograph) for a considerable length of time if the patient consumed a large volume of carbonated beverage before intubation

164. True statements regarding lasers include

    (1) the most serious danger during airway surgery with lasers is airway fire
    (2) if an airway fire occurs, recommended practice is to leave the endotracheal tube in place while the pharynx is flushed with saline
    (3) oxygen concentrations should not exceed 30% when laser surgery is performed in the facial area
    (4) some lasers can be damaging to the eyes; however, eyes are protected as long as normal eyeglasses are worn

165. A 70-kg healthy man received 80 mg succinylcholine for tracheal intubation. Which of the following modes of electric stimulation would be appropriate for monitoring the neuromuscular blockade?

    (1) Train-of-four before and after injection of succinylcholine
    (2) Posttetanic count at 50 Hz before and after injection of succinylcholine
    (3) Single twitch before and after injection of succinylcholine
    (4) Posttetanic count at 100 Hz before and after injection of succinylcholine

166. Which of the following will be seen during CVP monitoring?

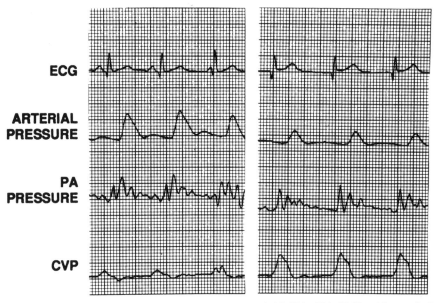

From Miller, *Anesthesia,* 3/e, and Sykes MK, *Br J Anaesth* 40:666–674, 1968, with permission.

(1)   Cannon *a* waves will be seen on the pressure tracing during atrial fibrillation
(2)   The *a* waves will be absent in nodal rhythms
(3)   The *y* descent will occur during tricuspid valve closure
(4)   Giant *v* waves may be present in tricuspid regurgitation

---

167. True statements regarding somatosensory evoked potentials (SSEPs) include

(1)   they monitor the integrity of motor pathways in anesthetized patients undergoing surgical procedures that place these pathways at risk
(2)   they negate the need for intraoperative "wake-up" tests
(3)   an increased amplitude and a decreased latency are common first signs of impaired blood flow to the spinal cord
(4)   they are prone to both false-positive and false-negative results when used during spinal surgery

168. The pressure gauge for oxygen on the anesthesia machine reads 45 PSIG. Which of the following measures should be taken immediately?

(1)   Check that the anesthesia machine is still connected to the central oxygen pipeline
(2)   Change the oxygen tank on the anesthesia machine because it is empty
(3)   Check that the central pipeline for oxygen is not malfunctioning and producing a lower reading on the pressure gauge
(4)   Check to make sure the central oxygen and nitrous oxide lines have not been crossed

169. True statements about modern vaporizers include

(1) they are the variable-bypass type
(2) carrier gas flows over vaporizing anesthetic
(3) they are out of circuit
(4) they are agent-specific

170. True statements regarding anesthesia equipment include

(1) assigning a classification of *semiopen, semiclosed,* or *closed* to a breathing system has to do with the degree of closure of the APL (pop-off) valve
(2) the main advantage of a Jackson-Rees circuit over a circle system for pediatric patients is its conservation of humidity
(3) the main advantage of a closed system is that there is no rebreathing
(4) the most efficient circle system for highest conservation of fresh gas has the inspiratory and expiratory valves as close to the patient as possible

171. True statements concerning anesthesia ventilators include

(1) the power source of the machine is pneumatic, electrical, or both
(2) compressed gases are the driving force of the bellows
(3) standing bellows are safer than hanging bellows
(4) the machines are pressure-cycled

172. True statements about the circle system include

(1) a semiopen system has no rebreathing of exhaled gases
(2) a semiclosed system has partial rebreathing of exhaled gases
(3) a closed system has total rebreathing of exhaled gases except for carbon dioxide
(4) there is poor conservation of heat and moisture in the circle system

173. True statements about anesthesia circuits include

(1) the expiratory valve of a circle system requires 2 to 3 cmH_2O pressure to open
(2) using the oxygen flush, approximately 50 L/min of gas can be delivered
(3) in many anesthesia machines, oxygen flushing can cause higher vaporizer output than appears on the dialed setting
(4) whether the oxygen flowmeter is upstream or downstream from the other flowmeters is not particularly important in the design of an anesthesia machine

174. Accurate descriptions of the Bain circuit include that it

(1) may lead to hypercarbia secondary to inadequate fresh gas flow
(2) does not allow for scavenging of waste gases
(3) has a coaxial circuit that allows warming of the inhaled fresh gas
(4) can only be used in a spontaneously breathing patient

MACHINERY

ANSWERS

129. **The answer is E.** (Miller, 4/e. p 189.) The "fail-safe" valve senses a drop in O_2 pressure as O_2 enters the anesthesia machine. It proportionately decreases the supply pressure of all other gases, including N_2O, to prevent delivery of a hypoxic mixture to the machine. However, this will not prevent hypoxic mixtures from being delivered to the patient if there are leaks or unlinked flowmeters. It also fails to protect against hypoxic mixtures if there has been a crossing of the N_2O and O_2 main supply lines.

130. **The answer is A.** (Miller, 4/e. p 2409.) Traditionally, ventilators are named by the parameter that ends the inspiratory phase of ventilation; thus, in a volume-cycled ventilator, preset volume determines the end of the inspiratory phase. The advantages of these ventilators include the fact that the volume of gas delivered to the patient is easy to control, volume delivery is not affected by pathophysiologic changes in the patient, and changes in airway pressure waveforms are easy to accomplish.

131. **The answer is E.** (Miller, 4/e. p 188.) The fail-safe valve is located in a manner that protects against both wall and cylinder reductions in O_2 pressure. Pin indexing is used on these tanks to ensure attachment of each gas to its proper pipeline. The flush valve will work with both wall supply and cylinder supply of O_2. The cylinders are indeed at a higher pressure than the wall supply (220 psi for O_2 and 745 psi for N_2O), but before entry into the machine, a pressure regulator decreases the total to 45 psi, lower than the wall pressure of 50 psi. There are times, such as during use of the oxygen flush valve, when pressure in the machine drops below 45 psi and causes slow depletion of the tanks. Therefore, they should be checked daily and kept closed unless needed.

132. **The answer is E.** (Miller, 4/e. p 188. Rogers, pp 967–970.) The color of an oxygen E cylinder is always green in the United States. The oxygen in the E cylinder is a compressed gas that is 2000 PSIG and contains approximately 625 L of oxygen. As the tank empties, pressure and the amount of oxygen are proportional; i.e., at 1000 PSIG, there will remain 312.5 L of oxygen. The E cylinder also contains a pressure reduction valve that reduces flow to a constant 45 to 50 PSIG.

133.   **The answer is A.** (Miller, 4/e. p 203.) Figure A is a Mapleson A system. During spontaneous ventilation, exhaled alveolar gas is released through the expiratory valve. During inspiration, fresh gas and dead space gas flow to the patient and do not contain carbon dioxide. Fresh gas flow need only equal the patient's minute ventilation. Disposition of gas at end-expiration is shown in circuits A through D, with spontaneous ventilation on the left and controlled ventilation on the right.

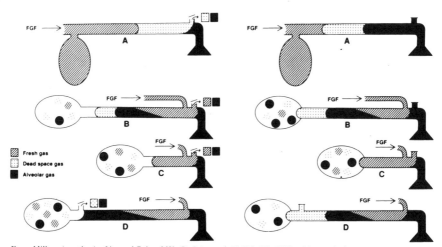

From Miller, *Anesthesia*, 3/e, and Sykes MK, *Br J Anaesth* 40:666–674, 1968, with permission.

134.   **The answer is E.** (Miller, 4/e. p 205.) This is a Bain circuit. It is a Mapleson D circuit modified so that the fresh gas flow is inside the corrugated tubing, which adds warmth and humidity to the inhaled gases. However, unless clear corrugated tubing is used, a disconnection within the tubing may go undetected. A fresh gas flow of 70 mL/kg is needed to prevent rebreathing during controlled ventilation, and 200 to 300 mL/kg is needed during spontaneous ventilation.

135.   **The answer is C.** (Rogers, p 971.) The color of an N_2O E cylinder is always blue in the United States. N_2O is in a compressed liquid phase until it exits the tank as a gas. A full N_2O E cylinder has 745 PSIG and contains 1600 L. Pressure left in the tank is not proportional to the amount of N_2O left in the tank. The pressure in an E cylinder will start to decrease only when the tank is 80 percent empty. A more accurate way to discern how many liters of N_2O is left in the tank is to weigh the tank. A full N_2O tank weighs 9.0 kg, and an empty tank weighs 6.0 kg; 1600 L of N_2O weighs 3.0 kg.

136. **The answer is D.** (Rogers, p 97.) A full E tank carries 659 L of oxygen; therefore, at 6 L/min, the tank will run out in 110 min.

137. **The answer is B.** (Miller, 4/e. p 1414.) "IT" refers to having passed tissue toxicity testing. It stands for "implant tested." The label "Z-79" on some endotracheal tubes stands for the same thing.

138. **The answer is D.** (Miller 4/e. p 1169.) The zero reference is at the stopcock that is opened to atmospheric pressure during calibration. Ideally, this should also be at the level of the right atrium. The transducer dome, which actually measures the blood pressure, should be at the level of the right atrium.

139. **The answer is D.** (Miller, 4/e. pp 1098, 1167–1168.) Air bubbles in the system will increase dampening of the waveform by increasing the elastic component of the system. Detail in the waveform can be lost with overdampening. Tubing diameter is a component of the formula for determining the "ring" frequency. Excessive "ringing" in the system occurs when the natural frequency of the system is too close to that of the blood pressure's signal, 20 Hz. Long tubing causes a drop in system frequency so that it approaches 20 Hz, which causes excessive ringing. Increasing the dampening can reduce ringing in a system. A small air bubble can be useful in reducing ringing when tubing must be long because it dampens the system.

140. **The answer is D.** (Miller, 4/e. p 1165.) The most common method is the oscillometric technique. Variations in cuff pressures during deflation are sensed and used for the determination of the arterial blood pressure.

141. **The answer is D.** (Miller, 4/e. pp 1264–1265.) Dyes can affect pulse oximetry: methylene blue > indocyanine green > indigo carmine > fluorescin. At high methemoglobin concentrations, Sa_{O_2} approaches 85 percent. Bright lights can cause falsely elevated Sa_{O_2}. Polycythemia has no effect on Sa_{O_2}.

142. **The answer is D.** (Miller, 4/e. pp 1357, 1346.) Administration of > 1 mg/kg of succinylcholine will abolish all twitches on train-of-four monitoring.

143. **The answer is B (1, 3).** (Miller, 4/e. pp 115–119.) If the inspired flow rate equals or is higher than the rate of ventilation, rebreathing is essentially abolished. Rebreathed gas has some amount of anesthetic gas removed from it, which makes prediction of the actual inspired concentration difficult. When rebreathing is eliminated, the predicted and actual inspired concentrations are the same. Rebreathing preserves the humidity of inspired gases; some rebreathed or alveolar gas is more humid than fresh gas. At high flow rates, rebreathing is reduced or eliminated.

144. **The answer is A (1, 2, 3).** (Miller, 4/e. pp 207–208.) Water used to promote the absorptive tendencies of soda lime for CO_2 actually comes from the patient. NaOH is the catalyst. The reaction is as follows:

$$CO_2 + H_2O \rightarrow H_2CO_3$$
$$H_2CO_3 + 2NaOH \rightarrow Na_2CO_3 + 2H_2O + heat$$
$$Na_2CO_3 + Ca(OH)_2 \rightarrow CaCO_3 + 2NaOH$$

145. **The answer is D (4).** (Miller, 4/e. p 1164.) Systolic point is determined as the pressure at which pulsations are increasing and are 25 percent and 50 percent of the maximum pulsations. Diastolic pressure is determined where pulsation amplitude has decreased to 80 percent of the maximum pulsation. The oscillometric method measures amplitudes of arterial pulsation. Maximum amplitude is read as mean arterial pressure. Systolic and diastolic pressures are derived from this.

146. **The answer is E (all).** (Miller, 4/e. pp 1163–1165.) Long stethoscope tubing can interfere with the transmission and interpretation of sounds, as can poor hearing. Korotkoff sounds are dependent on flow of blood. Decreased blood flow, such as that caused by shock or the use of vasopressors, can delay the transmission of sounds and cause underestimation of blood pressure.

147. **The answer is D (4).** (Miller, 4/e. pp 1163–1165.) Cuff width should be 20 to 30 percent of the limb circumference. Cuffs that are too wide will give artificially low blood pressures, while cuffs that are too narrow will give artificially high blood pressures. Deflation rate should be slow, about 3 mmHg/s, to allow sensors to pick up sounds. Otherwise, readings will be low. When atherosclerotic vessels underlie the cuff, because of low vessel compliance, high occlusion pressures are needed to occlude the vessels in order to hear Korotkoff sounds, which results in falsely elevated blood pressure.

148. **The answer is E (all).** (Miller, 4/e. pp 1164–1165.) All these problems have occurred with automated blood pressure devices. They are rare and usually are due to frequent inflation of the cuff.

149. **The answer is B (1, 3).** (Miller, 4/e. pp 1187–1188.) The thermal dilution technique of cardiac output measurements uses the difference in temperature between the blood and the injectate as the indicator. The thermistor in the pulmonary artery catheter acts as a variable resistor in a Wheatstone bridge, with a linear relationship between temperature and electrical resistance so that the output from the bridge is dependent on the change in temperature. Cardiac output is calculated by a computer. This technique measures the output from the right side of the heart. Inaccurate measurements may occur with intracardiac shunts and infusion of large volumes of fluids into the right side of the heart.

150. **The answer is B (1, 3).** (Miller, 4/e. pp 1186–1188.) Multiple measurements increase the confidence limits of the value significantly. Cold rather than room temperature injectates do not have a significant effect on the accuracy of the cardiac output measurements. Furthermore, iced injectates can cause dysrhythmias. Because respiration affects intrathoracic pressures and thus instantaneous cardiac outputs, it is best to measure outputs consistently in the same phase of respiration. The ECG phase does not affect measurement of cardiac output.

151. **The answer is A (1, 2, 3).** (Miller, 4/e. pp 1265–1266.) Mixed venous oxygen saturation is reflective of cardiac output when the oxygen supply and demand are relatively constant. It can be best appreciated by the following equation:

$$Sv_{O_2} = Sa_{O_2} - (V_{O_2}/CO \times Hb \times 1.34)$$

152. **The answer is C (2, 4).** (Miller, 4/e. pp 1199–1208.) The TEE has numerous diagnostic uses in the cardiac patient, including continuous monitoring of cardiac function, assessment of global and regional function, visualization of abnormal anatomy, and the ability to see intracardiac air emboli and perform contrast dye studies. It is limited by the subjectivity of the practitioner and is a highly sensitive, but not specific, marker of myocardial ischemia.

153. **The answer is E (all).** (Miller, 4/e. p 1185.) Careful use of PA catheters is necessary to prevent pulmonary artery rupture. Slow inflation of the balloon allows the inflation to sense vessel compliance and avoid balloon overinflation. Smaller vessels are at higher risk for rupture, and so if the catheter migrates, it should be pulled back. High balloon volumes increase the pressure on vessels and the risk of rupture. However, in the elderly, even low balloon pressures may cause rupture of pulmonary vessels.

154. **The answer is A (1, 2, 3).** (Miller, 4/e. pp 1199–1208.) The basic view of TEE does not visualize the right ventricular outflow tract, though portions of the right ventricle are visible.

155. **The answer is E (all).** (Miller, 4/e. pp 1177–1186.) PADP usually is an accurate indicator of PAOP. However, PADP is influenced by hypoxia, hyperthermia, and hypercarbia, all of which can raise PVR, the result of which will be a high PADP but a normal PAOP. Tachycardia decreases diastolic filling time, which may give a falsely elevated PADP.

156. **The answer is B (1, 3).** (Miller, 4/e. pp 1177–1180.) When properly placed, a PA catheter will stop phasic blood flow in the occluded pulmonary artery, which creates a static column of blood between the catheter tip and the left atrium. The catheter tip must be in zone III of the lung, where pulmonary venous pressure is greater than alveolar pressure. In zone II, alveolar pressure exceeds pulmonary venous pressure and PAOP will reflect alveolar pressure. In the normal heart, PAOP does give a good estimate of left atrial pressure. This in turn is a reflection of left ventricular end-diastolic pressure and volume (LVEDP and LVEDV). LVEDV is a good measure of preload. PEEP can close pulmonary vessels, which falsely elevates PA pressure measurements.

157. **The answer is D (4).** (Stoelting, *Pharmacology,* 2/e. p 694.) Left atrial filling occurs during ventricular systole, not diastole. The *v* wave occurs during ventricular systole, which, on the ECG tracing, follows the QRS complex and includes the T wave. The *c* wave is simultaneous with mitral valve closure and represents a transient increase in left atrial pressure as the mitral valve transiently bulges (because of left ventricular contraction) into the left atrium.

158. **The answer is E (all).** (Miller, 4/e. p 1177.) By definition, central venous pressure is the pressure measured at the junction of the vena cava and the right atrium. It is dependent on the intravascular volume and the vascular tone and can be used to measure both the right heart contractile function and filling force. Changes in intrathoracic pressure, such as those which occur during a ventilatory cycle, will be reflected in the pressure reading.

159. **The answer is D (4).** (Miller, 4/e. pp 1117–1119.) A maximal Sa_{O_2} of 100 percent occurs at P_{O_2} of approximately 100 torr; at a higher P_{O_2}, Sa_{O_2} does not change. Pulse oximeters measure the absorbance of 4 wavelengths of light. Functional and fractional oxygen saturation are two ways of measuring Sa_{O_2}, but neither way applies to the measurement made by pulse oximetry. Serum bilirubin does not affect Sa_{O_2}. Carboxyhemoglobin absorbs light in a fashion similar to that of oxyhemoglobin, and so a falsely high Sa_{O_2} occurs in the setting of a high carboxyhemoglobin level.

160. **The answer is D (4).** (Miller, 4/e. pp 1169–1170.) The Allen test is a poor predictor of ischemic complications after radial arterial cannulation. Ischemic complications from radial arterial cannulation have developed in patients with a normal Allen test. And in those with an abnormal Allen test, complications have not always occurred. Moreover, there is a poor correlation between a normal test and the presence of distal blood flow as assessed by injection of fluorescin dye.

161. **The answer is B (1, 3).** (Miller, 4/e. pp 1271–1274.) Obstruction to exhalation of CO_2 from the airways, as in bronchospasm or a kinked endotracheal tube, produces a less steep expiratory upstroke because CO_2 takes longer to reach the CO_2 detector. Both a large pulmonary embolus and severe bronchospasm will produce low end-tidal CO_2. In the case of a pulmonary embolus, this is due to increased dead-space ventilation; in the case of bronchospasm, it is due to inability of alveoli to empty through constricted airways. The inspiratory baseline is zero as long as inspired gases are devoid of CO_2. When inspired gases contain CO_2, as occurs when the CO_2 absorbent is exhausted, the inspiratory baseline will be elevated. Capnometers use infrared light to measure CO_2 absorption.

162. The answer is A (1, 2, 3). (Miller, 4/e. pp 1272–1273.) In the presence of a pulmonary embolus, areas of lung are ventilated but not perfused and there is no CO_2 transfer in those areas. Therefore, there is a dilution of the alveolar CO_2 with a resultant decrease in end-tidal CO_2.

163. The answer is B (1, 3). (Miller, 4/e. pp 1271–1274.) Elevated end-tidal CO_2 also can be caused by tourniquet release and hypermetabolic states such as malignant hyperthermia. Dead-space ventilation causes widening of the gradient of arterial to end-tidal CO_2 because alveoli that are ventilated but not perfused do not contain CO_2, and therefore the end-tidal CO_2 decreases (owing to the dilutional effect of air devoid of CO_2 passing by the CO_2 detector) while arterial CO_2 builds up (since the nonperfused lung cannot aid in CO_2 removal). However, when a shunt is present, alveoli that are perfused but not ventilated do not contribute CO_2 to end-tidal gases, while the blood that perfuses these alveoli builds up CO_2 (because CO_2 exchange does not take place here). When this blood, which contains an elevated CO_2 content, perfuses ventilated alveoli, the end-tidal CO_2 will reflect arterial CO_2; that is, it will be elevated. Therefore, both the arterial CO_2 and the end-tidal CO_2 will increase, but the difference will not change. The delivered tidal volume depends in part on the rate of fresh gas flow. Even without altering ventilatory settings, the effect of increasing fresh gas flow is delivery of a larger tidal volume, which results in an increased minute ventilation and a lowering of arterial as well as end-tidal CO_2. CO_2 in the stomach will quickly be washed away, and within a few breaths the CO_2 waveform will disappear.

164. The answer is B (1, 3). (Miller, 4/e. pp 2189–2190.) Endotracheal tubes can ignite, and so they should be removed promptly if an airway fire occurs, and the pharynx should then be flushed with saline. Special goggles appropriate to the type of laser used are necessary to protect the eyes of all operating room personnel. The patient's eyes should be taped closed and covered with moist gauze.

165. The answer is B (1, 3). (Miller, 4/e. pp 1346–1350.) A depolarizing neuromuscular block is characterized by a decrease in single-twitch height compared with control and by absence of fade to train-of-four or tetanic stimulation.

166. The answer is D (4). (Miller, 4/e. p 1177.) The *a* wave is caused by atrial contraction. It is therefore absent in atrial fibrillation. Cannon, or giant, *a* waves can be seen with nodal or heart block rhythms. They are caused by the contraction of the atrium against a closed tricuspid valve. The *y* descent occurs during opening of the tricuspid valve and ventricular filling. The *v* wave reflects the buildup of pressure as the right atrium fills. This can be magnified if there is tricuspid regurgitation.

167. The answer is D (4). (Miller, 4/e. pp 1329–1333.) SSEPs monitor the integrity of sensory pathways. They monitor pathways located dorsally in the spinal cord and may not detect anterior spinal cord injury involving motor fibers. A wake-up test, by assessing motor function, can reveal anterior spinal cord compromise. A decreased amplitude and an increased latency are early signs of ischemia. Localized anterior spinal cord ischemia can lead to false negatives, while interference of SSEPs by many factors, such as potent inhalational anesthetics, can cause false positives.

168. **The answer is B (1, 3).** (Miller, 4/e. p 188.) In some older anesthesia machines, the pipeline pressure gauge reading is on the machine side. Usually, the pipeline should read 50 PSIG, while tanks read 45 PSIG. Therefore, a lower reading of 45 PSIG may be due to central pipeline problems or a disconnection from the pipelines with the machine still connected to the tanks. Crossed gas lines will not affect the pressure reading.

169. **The answer is E (all).** (Miller, 4/e. pp 196–197.) *Variable bypass* means that the concentration of the final gas mixture depends on how much carrier gas bypasses the vaporizing chamber where anesthetic gas is picked up. The carrier gas flows over vaporizing anesthetic liquid and becomes saturated with it before leaving the vaporizer. The modern vaporizers are outside the breathing circuit. Vaporizers today are agent-specific and have a pin-indexing system to prevent filling with the wrong agent. Copper kettles were multi-agent.

170. **The answer is D (4).** (Miller, 4/e. pp 205–206.) Assignment of the terms *semiopen, semiclosed,* and *closed* to a system has to do with the absence or presence of rebreathing in the system and the amount of fresh gas inflow within the system. The Jackson-Rees circuit is more lightweight and portable, but it is less able to conserve humidity because a fresh gas flow rate of three times the patient's minute ventilation is required to prevent rebreathing. Other advantages over the circle system are lack of complexity, inexpensiveness, and lack of moving parts, which can cause resistance in the system. In a closed system, only the amount of fresh gas that is taken up by the patient need enter the system. Rebreathing is complete and therefore requires a method of efficiently absorbing carbon dioxide, such as soda lime or a mixture of barium and calcium hydroxide (Baralyme). Ideally, valves are close to the patient, but for ease of use, the inspiratory and expiratory valves are distant from the patient in all circle systems used today. This promotes mixing of alveolar and dead-space gases before they are vented.

171. **The answer is A (1, 2, 3).** (Miller, 4/e. pp 208–209.) During a disconnection, hanging bellows will continue to fill with entrained air from the site of disconnection, which prevents detection of the problem, while a standing bellows immediately collapses and makes the disconnection obvious. Anesthesia machines are time-cycled.

172. **The answer is A (1, 2, 3).** (Miller, 4/e. pp 206–207.) Flow rates determine whether a system is semiopen, semiclosed, or closed. Very high flow rates create a semiopen system, which prevents rebreathing. A closed system delivers gas at very low flow rates to exactly match the rate consumed by the patient. One of the advantages of the circle system is that there is excellent conservation of heat and moisture compared with other systems.

173. **The answer is A (1, 2, 3).** (Miller, 4/e. pp 192, 199, 202–203, 208–209.) In a circle system, 2 to 3 cmH$_2$O of positive end-expiratory pressure is built into the system. With an oxygen flush, 35 to 75 L/min is delivered. The higher vaporizer output with flushing is called the *pumping effect* and is due to retrograde pressure transmitted to the vaporizer, which promotes additional vaporizer output that moves in a retrograde direction and is suddenly released. The oxygen flowmeter should be downstream from all other flowmeters to help prevent delivery of a hypoxic mixture to the patient if there is a flowmeter leak.

174. **The answer is B (1, 3).** (Miller, 4/e. p 205.) The Bain circuit allows for scavenging of waste gases and can be used for controlled and spontaneous ventilation.

DISEASE STATES

Directions: Each question below contains four or five suggested responses. Select the **one best** response to each question.

175. An example of nociceptive pain is

  (A) pain from chronic degenerative joint disease
  (B) phantom limb pain
  (C) postherpetic neuralgia
  (D) refractory pain after spinal cord injury
  (E) refractory pain after cerebrovascular injury

176. A patient with renal failure has acute pain from a fractured femur. Which drug is contraindicated for pain control in this patient?

  (A) Morphine
  (B) Sufentanil
  (C) Hydromorphone
  (D) Meperidine
  (E) Fentanyl

177. A true statement about nonsteroidal anti-inflammatory drugs is

  (A) they work at both peripheral and central sites to block prostaglandin synthesis
  (B) they work primarily by stimulating the production of cyclooxygenase
  (C) the effect of aspirin on platelet function is reversed 24 h after discontinuing the drug
  (D) food ingestion with these drugs decreases their absolute bioavailability
  (E) in general, these drugs demonstrate very little protein binding

178. In prescribing medications for chronic pain,

    (A) nonnarcotic analgesics often can control pain of nonmalignant origin

    (B) drugs should be prescribed on a PRN (as circumstances require) basis

    (C) narcotics should be avoided because they are addictive

    (D) sedative-hypnotics such as benzodiazepines can be taken for a long time without the development of dependency

    (E) diphenhydramine and hydroxyzine are potentially addictive and should be avoided

179. The earliest sign in the development of malignant hyperthermia is

    (A) myoglobinuria
    (B) increased temperature
    (C) muscle rigidity
    (D) increased end-tidal CO_2
    (E) acidosis

Directions: Each question below contains four suggested responses of which **one or more** is correct. Select

(A)	if	**1, 2, and 3**	are correct
(B)	if	**1 and 3**	are correct
(C)	if	**2 and 4**	are correct
(D)	if	**4**	is correct
(E)	if	**1, 2, 3, and 4**	are correct

180. Disease states associated with airway abnormalities include

(1) Pierre Robin syndrome
(2) preeclampsia
(3) Treacher Collins syndrome
(4) gastroschisis

181. True statements in relation to patients with transplanted hearts include

(1) atherosclerosis of the donated heart is a frequent complication
(2) hepatic toxicity, usually manifested by elevated levels of transaminase, is the most common organ toxicity associated with use of cyclosporine
(3) azathioprine (Imuran) often causes leukopenia
(4) newer immunosuppressants, which have become the standard of care in these patients, have made opportunistic infections rare

182. True statements about the anesthesia physical status (PS or ASA) classification system include

(1) the higher the numerical assignment, the greater the anesthetic risk
(2) a healthy, normally functioning, 30-year-old person with morbid obesity should be designated class II
(3) a patient who presents for emergency coronary artery bypass graft, who is on an intraaortic balloon pump for refractory angina, and who has severe left main coronary artery disease should be designated class IV-E
(4) a patient with severe emphysema who requires home oxygen therapy to do light household work and who comes for elective herniorraphy should be designated class III

183. Cardiac transplantation is accurately characterized by which of the following statements?

- (1) Atropine, in usual doses, is the initial drug of choice in a cardiac transplant patient who becomes bradycardic intraoperatively
- (2) Vagal stimulation has more profound effects on heart rate in a cardiac transplant patient than in a normal patient
- (3) The peak vasopressor effect of ephedrine is more rapid in a cardiac transplant patient than in normal patients
- (4) Usual doses of antimuscarinic agents, such as atropine or glycopyrrolate, should be given to these patients when muscle relaxants are reversed with neostigmine or edrophonium

184. True statements about management of an asthmatic patient include

- (1) halothane is a better bronchodilating drug to use in asthmatic patients than the other halogenated volatile anesthetics
- (2) dexamethasone is not an effective intravenous steroid for the treatment of asthma
- (3) anticholinergic drugs cause mild increases in airway resistance and are ideally avoided in asthmatic patients
- (4) in trying to establish the severity of disease in a patient with asthma, a chest x-ray is not as useful as pulmonary function tests

185. Considerations in managing patients on antiasthma medication include

  (1) beta$_2$ agonists such as terbutaline protect against halothane-induced dysrhythmias
  (2) aminophylline treatment results in increased circulating norepinephrine
  (3) steroids will sensitize the myocardium to dysrhythmias
  (4) aminophylline may lower the ventricular fibrillation threshold

186. True statements regarding perioperative steroid coverage include which of the following?

  (1) Cardiovascular instability is a common problem in patients chronically on steroids who do not receive a stress dose in the preoperative or early intraoperative period
  (2) Patients who receive topical steroids need not be considered at risk for adrenal suppression since systemic absorption of steroids is minimal by this route
  (3) An appropriate recommendation for a patient chronically taking prednisone is for 500 mg hydrocortisone to be given IM every 8 h on the day of surgery for major operations
  (4) Hydrocortisone is slightly less potent than cortisol

187. Side effects of glucocorticoids include

  (1) thin skin and easy bruisability
  (2) decreased wound healing and increased infections
  (3) osteopenia and avascular necrosis
  (4) dehydration and hypotension

188. Drugs known to increase digoxin levels include

  (1) quinidine
  (2) hydrochlorothiazide
  (3) amiodarone
  (4) propranolol

189. Some neurologic diseases and their anesthetic implications include

  (1) in patients being treated for Parkinson's disease, droperidol probably should not be used
  (2) L-dopa, used for treatment of Parkinson's disease, can be arrhythmogenic
  (3) elevation of body temperature in patients with multiple sclerosis can aggravate symptoms of the disease
  (4) symptoms of multiple sclerosis can be exacerbated with use of spinal or epidural anesthesia

190. In patients with hypothyroidism,

  (1) minimum alveolar concentration (MAC) is decreased
  (2) there may be low voltage in the ECG
  (3) atrial fibrillation is a common finding
  (4) the stress response may be blunted

191. In anesthetizing patients who have received chemotherapy,

    (1)   folic acid analogues such as methotrexate can cause severe liver dysfunction

    (2)   anthracycline antibiotics such as doxorubicin can cause cardiomyopathies

    (3)   antineoplastic alkaloids such as vincristine can cause peripheral neuropathies and SIADH

    (4)   alkylating agents such as cyclophosphamide can prolong neuromuscular blockade

192. When one is anesthetizing patients with hyperthyroidism,

    (1)   sympathomimetic drugs should generally be avoided

    (2)   regional anesthesia should be avoided

    (3)   a thyroid storm may mimic malignant hyperthermia

    (4)   associated muscle rigidity may make patients resistant to muscle relaxants

193. With regard to adrenocortical insufficiency,

    (1)   signs and symptoms include darkened pigmentation, hyperkalemia, and hemoconcentration

    (2)   it may be diagnosed definitively by elevated ACTH levels

    (3)   patients manifest increased sensitivity to myocardial depressant drugs

    (4)   aldosterone secretion is abnormal in secondary adrenocortical insufficiency

194. True statements regarding hyperthyroidism include that it

    (1)   results in increased MAC

    (2)   results in increased oxygen consumption and heat production

    (3)   is associated with elevated plasma catecholamine levels

    (4)   makes the use of anticholinergic premedication unwise

195. With regard to patients with pheochromocytoma,

    (1)   alpha blockade is the first line of treatment

    (2)   the pheochromocytoma is under sympathetic nervous system control

    (3)   cardiomyopathy is secondary to catecholamine-induced myocardial necrosis

    (4)   pancuronium is the muscle relaxant of choice because it is excreted by both the kidneys and the liver

196. True statements about morbid obesity include which of the following:

    (1)   Blood pressures taken by cuffs of average size on obese extremities will register artificially low readings

    (2)   Even after careful denitrogenation, morbidly obese patients exhibit early oxygen desaturation primarily as a result of their high closing volumes

    (3)   Morbidly obese patients are at increased risk for pulmonary aspiration because they have a slower than normal gastric emptying time

    (4)   Cardiac output is elevated in these patients because of increased stroke volumes

197. Issues to be considered in cirrhotic patients include that

   (1) their volume of distribution is decreased

   (2) their glucose metabolism may be abnormal

   (3) hypoxemia is primarily due to progressive restrictive pulmonary disease

   (4) an elevated prothrombin time usually cannot be corrected by administration of vitamin K

198. Anesthetic considerations in alcoholic patients include

   (1) a cross tolerance for barbiturates, benzodiazepines, and alcohol

   (2) blood glucose monitoring is an important aspect of anesthetic management in an alcoholic patient who is receiving a general anesthetic

   (3) delirium tremens most often occurs 48 to 72 h after abstinence from alcohol

   (4) disulfiram may decrease sensitivity to anesthetic drugs

SUMMARY OF DIRECTIONS

A	B	C	D	E
1,2,3 only	1,3 only	2,4 only	4 only	All are correct

199. True statements regarding pulmonary aspiration include which of the following?

(1) Metoclopramide is an antidopaminergic drug that reduces lower esophageal sphincter pressure, increases gastric emptying, and reduces nausea

(2) The following are associated with an increased risk of pulmonary aspiration: emergency operations, repeated, failed endotracheal intubations, and airway trauma

(3) The three most important factors in determining the severity of pulmonary aspiration of gastric contents are pH of contents, volume of contents, and particulate versus nonparticulate nature of contents

(4) An adverse effect of H_2 blockers such as ranitidine and cimetidine is their stimulation of the mixed function oxidase system, which can result in unexpectedly low levels of propranolol

200. True statements about patients with advanced rheumatoid arthritis include

(1) symptoms of carpal tunnel syndrome occur after radial arterial lines

(2) to preserve cervical spine stability, the patient's neck should be maintained in the flexed position because extension can lead to spinal cord or medullary compression

(3) aspirin and corticosteroids, two agents used in the treatment of the disease, both have important implications for the anesthesiologist

(4) spinal anesthesia is contraindicated because the lumbar spine is usually affected by the disease

201. True statements about cardiac testing include which of the following?

(1) Cardiac catheterization is the gold standard for the diagnosis of coronary artery disease and estimation of left ventricular function

(2) In exercise stress testing, a drop of >10 mm Hg in systolic blood pressure suggests a low risk of heart disease

(3) Dipyridamole-thallium testing shows filling defects in areas of stenotic vessels on early images but reperfusion of these areas on late images

(4) Ejection fraction is equal to end-systolic volume (ESV) minus end-diastolic volume (EDV) divided by ESV; i.e., $(ESV - EDV)/ESV$

202. Important considerations in poorly controlled, chronically hypertensive patients include that

(1)　intraoperatively, blood pressure responses to sympathetic stimulation tend to be blunted

(2)　left ventricular hypertrophy with strain on ECG is not particularly helpful in assessing the severity of the disease

(3)　the cerebral autoregulatory curve is shifted to the left

(4)　the risk of myocardial infarction, stroke, arrhythmias, and congestive heart failure is increased

203. Signs and symptoms of anaphylaxis include

(1)　bronchospasm and airway edema

(2)　vasodilation and decreases in cardiac contractility

(3)　urticaria, erythema, and edema

(4)　severe systemic hypertension

204. Which of the following agents would be effective in the prevention of an anaphylactoid reaction from intravenous contrast dye?

(1)　Diphenhydramine

(2)　Ranitidine

(3)　Corticosteroids

(4)　Thiopental

205. In a patient who is being treated for myasthenia gravis, signs of a cholinergic crisis include

(1)　muscle weakness

(2)　dry mouth

(3)　bradycardia

(4)　improvement in muscle strength

206. The treatment regimen for organophosphate overdose may include

(1)　support of ventilation and hemodynamics

(2)　administration of atropine for the muscarinic effects

(3)　seizure prophylaxis with benzodiazepines

(4)　administration of pralidoxime for the nicotinic effects

207. Sequelae of an acute cocaine overdose include

(1)　myocardial ischemia and high-output cardiac failure

(2)　seizure activity

(3)　tremulousness and hyperthermia

(4)　decreased MAC

208. Carbon monoxide (CO) may be characterized by which of the following statements?

(1)　Poisoning results in increased minute ventilation

(2)　CO has twice the affinity for hemoglobin that oxygen has

(3)　CO shifts the oxyhemoglobin dissociation curve to the right

(4)　CO produces carboxyhemoglobin that absorbs the same frequency of light as oxyhemoglobin

209. In patients with carbon monoxide (CO) poisoning,

(1)　carboxyhemoglobin (COHb) is greater than 20%

(2)　pulse oximetry is a reliable measure of COHb

(3)　the half-life of COHb in room air is 5 h

(4)　hyperbaric O_2 is the treatment of choice

210. True statements concerning carbon monoxide (CO) poisoning include

(1) blood gases show normal Pa_{CO_2} and Pa_{O_2}, metabolic acidosis, and low oxygen saturations of hemoglobin

(2) hypoxia is caused by the strong affinity of CO for hemoglobin

(3) tissue hypoxia is caused by a shift to the left of the oxygen dissociation curve by carboxyhemoglobin

(4) there is a direct toxic effect on aerobic metabolic pathways

211. A 13-year-old black male with a family history of malignant hyperthermia is scheduled for cholecystectomy. Drugs likely to be associated with complications in this patient include

(1) atropine
(2) succinylcholine
(3) lidocaine
(4) halothane

212. Increased susceptibility to malignant hyperthermia is associated with

(1) Duchenne muscular dystrophy
(2) central core disease
(3) myopathy of unknown etiology
(4) cerebral palsy

SUMMARY OF DIRECTIONS

A	B	C	D	E
1,2,3	1,3	2,4	4	All are
only	only	only	only	correct

213. True statements regarding malignant hyperthermia (MH) include

(1) the absence of an elevated preoperative CPK in a patient with a family history of MH effectively rules out the disease in that patient

(2) nitrous oxide and droperidol are both safe drugs to use in patients with a history of MH

(3) dantrolene should be given preoperatively to all patients with a history of MH because it is more effective in preventing an MH response than in treating one

(4) the halothane/caffeine contracture test is both sensitive and specific for the diagnosis of MH

214. True statements regarding dantrolene include

(1) its action involves calcium flux

(2) its site of action is the sarcoplasmic reticulum

(3) an ampule of dantrolene also contains mannitol

(4) it alters neuromuscular transmission and electrical properties of skeletal muscle membranes

215. Dantrolene is correctly characterized by which of the following statements?

(1) It is associated with skeletal muscle weakness

(2) It is associated with hepatitis in patients receiving prolonged therapy

(3) It works directly on muscle fibrils

(4) It is used to treat neuroleptic malignant syndrome

216. True statements regarding neuroleptic malignant syndrome (NMS) include that

(1) it is due to aberrant calcium regulation

(2) its presence in a patient's history necessitates avoiding known triggering agents of malignant hyperthermia

(3) it is inherited

(4) it is treated with dantrolene symptomatically

217. Important considerations for patients with serious burn injuries include which of the following?

(1) In the first 24 h after the burn, patients should be given fluid at approximately 8 mL/kg per hour for each percent of body area burned

(2) Patients are resistant to nondepolarizing muscle relaxants primarily because the volume of distribution for these drugs is vastly increased

(3) Patients have a decreased requirement for opioids

(4) Patients do not respond normally to succinylcholine and may suffer cardiac arrest

218. True statements regarding burn patients include that they

   (1) may safely receive succinylcholine 28 to 35 days after the injury

   (2) show an increased resistance to depolarizing muscle relaxants

   (3) have an elevated plasma albumin concentration

   (4) may safely receive inhaled anesthetics

219. True statements regarding tricyclic antidepressants include that they

   (1) have anticholinergic effects

   (2) block the antihypertensive effects of clonidine

   (3) increase the requirements for inhalational anesthetics

   (4) can cause an exaggerated hypertensive response to direct-acting sympathomimetic drugs

220. In treating patients who have received phenothiazine drugs for a long period,

   (1) dopamine is the drug of choice for hypotension

   (2) significant beta blockade may be seen

   (3) there is a decreased sensitivity to narcotics and barbiturates

   (4) seizure threshold is lowered

221. True statements regarding monoamine oxidase (MAO) inhibitors include that they

   (1) are associated with hepatotoxicity

   (2) result in orthostatic hypotension

   (3) may result in hyperthermia when used in conjunction with opioids

   (4) result in increased requirements for inhaled anesthetics

222. In the anesthetic management of patients treated with MAO inhibitors,

   (1) most narcotics are safe to use

   (2) direct-acting sympathomimetic drugs can give an exaggerated response

   (3) indirect-acting sympathomimetic drugs should be used

   (4) regional blocks for pain control are probably safe to use

223. Lithium is accurately characterized by which of the following statements?

   (1) It is eliminated primarily via the kidneys

   (2) Levels are increased by furosemide

   (3) It prolongs the action of nondepolarizing muscle relaxants

   (4) It may increase inhaled anesthetic requirement

224. True statements about acute pain control include

   (1) transcutaneous electrical nerve stimulation (TENS) is thought to work by stimulating inhibitory dorsal horn neurons

   (2) local anesthetics are thought to work by complete blockade of neuronal transmission

   (3) Patient-controlled anesthesia (PCA) is thought to work by producing steady levels of drug without the wide swings in peaks and troughs seen with intermittent boluses

   (4) intrathecal narcotics are thought to work by modulating supraspinal opioid receptor sites and suppressing nociceptive reception in the spinal cord

225. True statements about neurolytic nerve blocks include

(1) they should be used only to treat pain of malignancy
(2) peripheral nerve destruction can result in denervation dysesthetic pain
(3) the blocks should be preceded by diagnostic nerve blocks
(4) neurolytic agents selectively destroy sensory tissue

226. True statements about causalgia include

(1) pain usually starts months after the injury has occurred
(2) pain is limited to the immediate area of injury
(3) pain is unaffected by stimulation of the sympathetic nervous system
(4) injury leading to causalgia is usually to major nerve trunks

227. True statements about reflex sympathetic dystrophy (RSD) include

(1) autonomic effects include changes in skin temperature, edema, and hyperhydrosis
(2) dystrophic changes include bone demineralization and stiff, painful joints
(3) surgery can trigger the syndrome
(4) hypalgesia is a common manifestation

228. Central pain or deafferentation pain states

(1) respond well to nonnarcotic analgesics
(2) respond well to narcotics
(3) usually respond to sedative hypnotics, at least for a short time
(4) respond best to phenytoin or carbamazepine

SUMMARY OF DIRECTIONS

A	B	C	D	E
1,2,3 only	1,3 only	2,4 only	4 only	All are correct

229. Aminophylline is characterized by which of the following descriptions?

   (1) It easily crosses the placenta

   (2) It may result in increased ventricular ectopy when used with halothane

   (3) It increases cardiac output and decreases peripheral vascular resistance

   (4) Its metabolism is slowed in cigarette smokers

230. Considerations in managing patients on antiasthma medication include

   (1) $beta_2$ stimulators such as terbutaline protect against halothane-induced dysrhythmias

   (2) aminophylline-type drugs result in increased circulating catecholamines

   (3) steroids will sensitize the myocardium to dysrhythmias

   (4) aminophylline may lower the ventricular fibrillation threshold

231. Lower esophageal sphincter (LES) tone is increased by

   (1) succinylcholine

   (2) atropine

   (3) metoclopramide

   (4) thiopental

232. True statements regarding carcinoid syndrome include

   (1) histamine release secondary to curare administration is detrimental

   (2) intraoperative bronchospasm is best treated with epinephrine

   (3) somatostatin will inhibit the release of vasoactive substances from carcinoid tumors

   (4) more than 50 percent of patients with carcinoid tumors will manifest carcinoid syndrome

DISEASE STATES

ANSWERS

175. **The answer is A.** (Miller, 4/e. p 2346.) Nociceptive pain is initiated by a peripheral receptor that sends signals to the dorsal horn of the spinal cord. The signal is passed through ascending tracts to cortical and subcortical sites. This nociceptive activation is caused by the detection of threatened or actual tissue damage in the periphery. All the other pains listed are examples of deafferentation pain in which the stimulus that produces the pain is thought to originate in the CNS.

176. **The answer is D.** (Barash, 3/e. p 953.) Meperidine has an active metabolite, normeperidine, that can accumulate in patients with renal failure. At high concentrations, this metabolite may cause CNS excitation. Its half-life is 12 to 16 h in people with normal renal function.

177. **The answer is A.** (Barash, 3/e. p 1313.) All the nonsteroidal anti-inflammatory drugs work both peripherally and centrally, although some, such as ketorolac, have far more central effects than peripheral effects. Many of the drugs in this group block the production of cyclooxygenase, a critical enzyme in prostaglandin synthesis. Platelet function is irreversible after aspirin ingestion. Food ingestion may slow the absorption of these drugs but not their absolute bioavailability, and they are highly protein bound.

178. **The answer is A.** (Miller, 4/e. pp 2348–2350.) There has been much abuse of drugs for chronic pain and poor judgment in their prescription. Nonnarcotic analgesics often can control pain that is not malignant in origin. They should be taken on a regular schedule rather than PRN so that pain does not have a chance to develop. A regular schedule usually results in less medication. Narcotics are addictive, but there are some patients, particularly those with terminal cancer, for whom opiates are the most effective therapy. The sedative effects of barbiturates and benzodiazepines are of short duration, and patients quickly need higher doses, which results in dependence. Diphenhydramine and hydroxyzine do not lead to dependence or withdrawal symptoms.

179. **The answer is D.** (Miller, 4/e. pp 1084–1086.) The earliest sign of increased metabolism resulting from malignant hyperthermia is an increase in end-expired CO_2 during constant ventilation. All the other signs are late manifestations.

180. **The answer is A (1, 2, 3).** (Stoelting, *Anesthesia and Co-Existing Disease,* 3/e. pp 564, 575, 596, 605.) Pierre Robin syndrome is characterized by micrognathia (small mouth) and glossoptosis (protruding tongue). The primary reason for airway difficulty in patients with preeclampsia is laryngeal and oropharyngeal edema. Mucosal fragility is another feature that may make airway management difficult. Children with Treacher Collins syndrome have micrognathia and often a cleft palate. Gastroschisis is rarely associated with other abnormalities. Omphalocele, by contrast, has a high association of other abnormalities, including macroglossia.

181. **The answer is B (1, 3).** (Stoelting, *Pharmacology,* 2/e. p 233.) Up to 50 percent of these patients develop atherosclerosis within 5 years of transplantation regardless of the age of the transplanted heart. Angina is rare because of denervation of the heart. Renal toxicity is the most common side effect of cyclosporine. These patients are markedly immunocompromised, and strict sterile technique should be observed for every invasive procedure.

182. **The answer is E (all).** (Miller, 4/e. pp 809–810.) Morbid obesity is accompanied by significant alterations in cardiopulmonary and gastrointestinal physiology that must be considered systemic disturbances. If the patient is otherwise healthy, a classification of class II is suitable. The patient in choice 3 has a life-threatening systemic disturbance and requires emergency surgery; this is best designated class IV-E. The patient in choice 4 has a severe systemic disturbance that interferes with normal activity but is not acutely life-threatening, and so a class III designation is appropriate.

183. **The answer is D (4).** (Barash, 3/e. pp 1271–1272. Stoelting, *Pharmacology,* 2/e. p 233.) The vagus is not connected to the transplanted heart; therefore, vagal tone does not affect heart rate, nor does atropine. Elevated heart rates can be achieved via beta agonists such as isoproterenol. Drugs with primarily indirect effects, such as ephedrine, take longer to act because of sympathetic denervation of the heart. Vasopressor effects require release of norepinephrine from intact sympathetic nerve endings followed by transport via the circulation of the heart, where direct alpha and beta agonism can take place. Although cardiac muscarinic effects are unlikely with anticholinesterase drugs in a patient with a transplanted heart, pulmonary and gastrointestinal muscarinic effects do occur and should be blocked with antimuscarinic agents.

184. **The answer is D (4).** (Stoelting, *Pharmacology,* 2/e. pp 200–202.) Halogenated volatile anesthetics are equieffective at bronchodilation. Halothane sensitizes the myocardium to the arrhythmogenic effects of sympathomimetics and therefore might be avoided in favor of isoflurane or enflurane. All steroids are effective in equipotent doses. Anticholinergic drugs decrease airway resistance and may therefore be beneficial. However, a potentially harmful effect of these drugs is that they may increase viscosity of airway secretions. A chest x-ray may be useful in showing a concomitant infectious process, but there are no specific radiographic findings in asthma. Certain of the pulmonary function tests, however, such as forced expiratory volume in 1 s (FEV_1) and maximal midexpiratory flow rate (MMEFR), will define the severity of disease.

185. **The answer is C (2, 4).** (Miller, 4/e. pp 992–993.) Even the $beta_2$ selective drugs, such as terbutaline, have some $beta_1$ activity. Dysrhythmias can occur, especially when high doses of these drugs are used. Xanthine drugs, such as aminophylline, are beta stimulators, which release norepinephrine and prevent the breakdown of cAMP by phosphodiesterase. The increased circulating catecholamines may cause dysrhythmias, especially in the presence of halothane. Xanthines do decrease the ventricular fibrillation threshold. Steroids have no effect on myocardial irritability.

186. **The answer is D (4).** (Stoelting, *Pharmacology,* 2/e. p 492.) Cardiovascular instability is actually an uncommon problem, but acute adrenal insufficiency can be catastrophic, and so many practitioners treat most, if not all, patients chronically taking steroids to avoid this complication. All forms of steroid therapy, including skin creams and ointments, can suppress normal adrenal responsiveness. The maximal dose secreted by the adrenals at times of maximal stress is 200 to 500 mg/day of cortisol (hydrocortisone 250 to 650 mg equivalent). Most authors recommend not more than 250 mg of hydrocortisone on the day of surgery with a taper to follow. Cortisone 25 mg is equivalent to cortisol 20 mg.

187. **The answer is A (1, 2, 3).** (Miller, 4/e. pp 916–921.) High levels of glucocorticoids are usually due to exogenous administration. The patients most likely to receive steroids include those with asthma, arthritis, or allergies. Fluid retention, hypertension, diabetes mellitus, psychoses, and muscle wasting are other side effects that are often seen. Studies disagree about whether any of these problems occur regularly after short courses of therapy. Topical vitamin A may reverse poor wound healing by stabilizing lysosomes.

188. **The answer is B (1, 3).** (Stoelting, *Pharmacology,* 2/e. pp 291–292, 350–351.) Quinidine and amiodarone both increase serum digoxin levels, which may lead to toxicity. Hydrochlorothiazide may lead to dig toxicity by reducing potassium levels but not by raising digoxin levels. Propranolol has no effect on dig levels.

189. **The answer is A (1, 2, 3).** (Stoelting, *Anesthesia and Co-Existing Disease,* 3/e. pp 209–211, 215–217.) Droperidol is a butyrophenone derivative which can exacerbate extrapyramidal symptoms in patients with Parkinson's disease being treated with L-dopa. Arrhythmia can also occur with L-dopa. For this reason, use of other drugs that promote dysrhythmias, such as halothane, should be avoided. In multiple sclerosis, demyelinated neurons that are barely functioning can cease conduction of nerve impulses when a rise in body temperature occurs. Spinal anesthesia has been implicated in postoperative exacerbations of symptoms in multiple sclerosis. This is thought to be due to neurotoxicity from local anesthetics. Epidural anesthesia has not been associated with these problems.

190. The answer is C (2, 4). (Barash, 3/e. pp 1042–1043.) There is no change in MAC unless hypothermia is present, in which case MAC is decreased. Atrial fibrillation is a feature of hyperthyroidism. Cholesterol-rich pericardial fluid may cause low voltage on the ECG. Resting cortisol levels are usually normal, but in long-standing disease there may be an ablated stress response.

191. The answer is E (all). (Miller, 4/e. pp 986–987.) The preoperative workup of cancer patients should include chemotherapeutic regimens. Folic acid analogues such as methotrexate may cause severe liver dysfunction. Anthracycline antibiotics such as doxorubicin can cause severe cardiomyopathies. Alkylating agents such as cyclophosphamide may cause thrombocytopenia, which precludes regional techniques, and may act as cholinesterase inhibitors, prolonging neuromuscular blockade.

192. The answer is B (1, 3). (Stoelting, *Anesthesia and Co-Existing Disease,* 3/e. pp 347–351.) Patients with hyperthyroidism generally show signs of increased sympathetic activity. They can be tachycardic and hyperthermic and can have atrial fibrillation, tremors, and skeletal muscle weakness. Beta blockers are part of standard treatment regimens. Regional anesthesia, with its associated sympathetic blockade, is a good choice as long as hemodynamic stability is maintained. Patients are often sensitive to muscle relaxants with a prolonged response.

193. The answer is B (1, 3). (Stoelting, *Anesthesia and Co-Existing Disease,* 3/e. pp 360–362.) Other symptoms of adrenocortical insufficiency include muscle weakness, weight loss, and hypoglycemia. ACTH levels will be elevated only in primary adrenocortical insufficiency. Patients with untreated hypoadrenocorticism are very sensitive to myocardial depressants. Aldosterone secretion remains normal in secondary adrenocortical insufficiency.

194. The answer is C (2, 4). (Stoelting, *Anesthesia and Co-Existing Disease,* 3/e. pp 347–351.) MAC is unchanged in hyperthyroidism, although increased cardiac output slows induction. Plasma catecholamine levels are not elevated. Anticholinergic premedication may increase heart rate and interfere with temperature regulation.

195. The answer is B (1, 3). (Stoelting, *Anesthesia and Co-Existing Disease,* 3/e. pp 363–367.) Alpha blockade is the first line of defense in patients with pheochromocytomas. This blocks vasoconstriction, decreasing blood pressure, and allows for volume repletion. Subsequent beta blockade may be necessary in patients with dysrhythmias. While a pheochromocytoma is derived from sympathetic tissue, it is not under sympathetic control but secretes secondarily to mechanical or pharmacologic stimuli. As a sympathetic stimulator, pancuronium is a poor choice because it may raise blood pressure.

196. The answer is D (4). (Barash, 3/e pp 975–976, 979.) Artificially high readings will be seen because the cuff has to inflate to abnormally high pressures (because of an excessively thick tissue layer over the artery) to effect arterial occlusion. Morbidly obese patients become hypoxic quickly because of a low functional residual capacity (which means a low oxygen reserve) and a high oxygen consumption caused by the increased body mass. In morbidly obese patients, gastric emptying is not slowed and may be hastened. Aspiration is a risk because of the prevalence of hiatal hernias and increased intra-abdominal pressures. Morbidly obese patients have elevated blood volumes, and cardiac output increases by 20 to 30 mL/min for each kilogram of adipose tissue. Hypertension and left ventricular hypertrophy are compensatory responses to chronically elevated stroke volumes.

197. **The answer is C (2, 4).** (Barash, 3/e. pp 1005–1007.) The volume of distribution is usually increased in cirrhotic patients. Increased plasma fatty acids interfere with the effect of insulin on glucose uptake. Increases in growth hormone and glucagon also interfere with carbohydrate metabolism. Hypoxia is common but is due to intrapulmonary shunting and basilar atelectasis. Ascites will cause basilar atelectasis and an increase in closing volume. Contributions to hypoxia also come from increased 2,3-diphosphoglycerate with a right shift of the oxyhemoglobin dissociation curve, hypoventilation, and an increase in closing volume, and an increase in closing volume. Diffusing capacity derangements can also occur. An elevated prothrombin time in advanced liver disease indicates the failure to synthesize coagulation factor, and vitamin K will not correct this defect. Fresh-frozen plasma is the treatment of choice in this situation.

198. **The answer is A (1, 2, 3).** (Stoelting, *Anesthesia and Co-Existing Disease*, 3/e. pp 526–528.) Many neurologic sequelae of alcohol abuse may be due to the effects on GABA receptors. There is an increase in GABA-mediated chloride ion conductance, an effect shared by benzodiazepines and barbiturates. Alcoholics are prone to hypoglycemia, and so blood glucose monitoring should be done routinely in anesthetized patients. Hypoglycemia is one etiology of alcohol-induced seizures. Delirium tremens should be considered whenever sympathetic hyperactivity, seizures, or hallucinations occur in the perioperative period. The condition may be masked by general anesthesia, and benzodiazepines should be administered whenever the diagnosis is suspected. Disulfiram, which prevents the full metabolism of alcohol, can cause sedation and may interfere with metabolism of other anesthetic drugs. This can potentiate anesthetic effects.

199. **The answer is A (1, 2, 3).** (Barash, 3/e. pp 1293–1294, 1144.) Metoclopramide has no effect on gastric acid pH but can be used effectively for aspiration prophylaxis in cases where delayed gastric emptying is an issue, such as pregnancy and diabetes mellitus. Patients at both extremes of age are at highest risk for pulmonary aspiration. All the other situations mentioned also predispose to pulmonary aspiration. Additional predisposing factors are a poor level of consciousness (such as ethanol intoxication), esophageal pathology or difficulty swallowing (such as amyotrophic lateral sclerosis or scleroderma), gastroesophageal junction incompetence (such as hiatal hernia), delayed gastric emptying (such as with analgesics or bowel obstruction), and elevated intragastric pressure (such as with ascites). A pH < 2.5 and volumes of 0.4 to 1 mL/kg can cause destruction of surfactant with alveolar collapse and capillary damage, which results in bronchospasm, ventilation-perfusion mismatch, and loss of lung volume. The presence of particulate matter can cause a granulomatous reaction in the lungs or airway obstruction with postobstructive infection. H_2 blockers inhibit the mixed function oxidase system, which results in unexpectedly high levels of the listed drugs (cimetidine has more of this effect than does ranitidine).

200.   The answer is B (1, 3). (Miller, 4/e. p 2126.) These patients are at high risk for carpal tunnel syndrome, which can be exacerbated after arterial lines in the wrist. Neck flexion should be avoided to maintain cervical spine stability; overflexion can lead to spinal cord or medullary compression. Awake intubation and positioning should be considered. Patients on aspirin have impaired platelet aggregation and clotting ability; patients on corticosteroids may require additional doses perioperatively to avoid adrenal insufficiency. They may also be at increased risk for ischemic heart disease. The lumbar spine is rarely affected by rheumatoid arthritis. Regional anesthesia is often a good choice.

201.   The answer is B (1, 3). (Miller, 4/e. pp 940–944.) Ejection fraction is derived from (EDV− ESV)/EDV. A normal value is 55 to 75 percent. During exercise stress testing a drop of SBP >10 mmHg, a low achieved heart rate, and an increase in diastolic blood pressure to >110 mmHg are all predictive of multivessel disease. Dipyridamole dilates normal vessels but does not affect stenotic vessels. Thallium imaging will reveal filling defects in the stenotic areas, followed by reperfusion after dilation has resolved.

202.   The answer is D (4). (Miller, 4/e. p 717.) Vascular hyperreactivity accompanied by heightened blood pressure responses occurs in these patients. Left ventricular hypertrophy on ECG indicates severe long-standing disease and a significant degree of left ventricular dysfunction. The cerebral autoregulatory curve is shifted to the right; higher blood pressures must be maintained to preserve cerebral perfusion.

203.   The answer is A (1, 2, 3). (Miller, 4/e. p 962.) Anaphylaxis is defined as an allergic reaction that may be life-threatening. It is mediated by IgE with release of vasoactive substances that are responsible for the typical end-organ responses. The response of the respiratory system results in bronchospasm and airway edema. In the cardiovascular system there may be precipitous decreases in cardiac output because of dilation of the capillaries and postcapillary venules. This leads to decreases in venous return, systemic vascular resistance, and edema. The vasoactive mediators also may directly reduce inotropy. Hypertension usually is not seen.

204.   The answer is A (1, 2, 3). (Miller, 4/e. p 962.) Numerous drugs can cause anaphylactoid reactions. Intravenous contrast dyes give the highest incidence. Patients who are at risk may be pretreated. Diphenhydramine is an H_1 blocker, and ranitidine is an H_2 blocker. These drugs may prevent the characteristic bronchospasm, venodilation, decrease in systemic vascular resistance, and edema that can occur. Corticosteroids may stabilize mast cells and basophils, which are responsible for the release of histamine and other vasoactive substances. Hydration is also recommended to counteract venodilation. Thiopental can initiate an anaphylactoid reaction and is not effective in prevention.

205.   The answer is B (1, 3). (Stoelting, *Anesthesia and Co-Existing Disease*, 3/e. p 441.) Anticholinesterase drugs (neostigmine and pyridostigmine) are used in the treatment of myasthenia gravis. These drugs are effective because they inhibit acetylcholinesterase, which is the enzyme responsible for the breakdown of acetylcholine. When a patient has had a relative overdose of an anticholinesterase drug, a cholinergic crisis may ensue with signs and symptoms that mimic worsening myasthenia. These include muscle weakness (nicotinic) and bradycardia, miosis, and salivation (muscarinic). If an intravenous dose of edrophonium 1 to 2 mg (Tensilon test) is given and the nicotinic and muscarinic effects worsen, the diagnosis is confirmed.

206. **The answer is E (all).** (Stoelting, *Anesthesia and Co-Existing Disease,* 3/e. pp 535–536.) Organophosphates cause phosphorylation of cholinesterase enzymes, which inactivates those enzymes and allows a buildup of acetylcholine. The phosphorylation reaction is reversible within 24 h if the antidote pralidoxime is given. Pralidoxime is a direct antagonist of the organophosphate. Once the antidote is given, acetylcholine will once again be broken down and symptoms will dissipate.

207. **The answer is A (1, 2, 3).** (Stoelting, *Anesthesia and Co-Existing Disease,* 3/e. pp 528–529.) Acute cocaine overdose will actually cause an increase in MAC because central catecholamine levels are increased. Cocaine inhibits the reuptake of norepinephrine. Increased circulating norepinephrine levels have numerous effects on the cardiac system, including coronary artery vasospasm, an increase in myocardial oxygen consumption, and an increase in systemic vascular resistance. These effects can cause high-output cardiac failure and cardiac ischemia.

208. **The answer is D (4).** (Stoelting, *Anesthesia and Co-Existing Disease,* 3/e. p 536.) Carotid and aortic bodies increase minute ventilation in response to a decreased Pa_{O_2}, not decreased hemoglobin saturation. Carbon monoxide has over 200 times the affinity for hemoglobin that oxygen has. Carboxyhemoglobin shifts the oxyhemoglobin dissociation curve to the left. Because carboxyhemoglobin absorbs the same frequency of light as oxyhemoglobin, oxyhemoglobin saturation may be overestimated in the presence of CO poisoning.

209. **The answer is B (1, 3).** (Miller, 4/e. pp 2431–2432.) Carbon monoxide is normally present and bound to about 1 percent of oxygen binding sites on hemoglobin. When a person is exposed to smoke, CO concentrations can rise dramatically; 20% defines poisoning. Because CO has 200 times greater affinity for hemoglobin than oxygen and is slow to be released, hypoxia can result. COHb and hemoglobin have similar absorption characteristics. Therefore, pulse oximetry will not give a reliable measure of COHb, overestimating the amount of hemoglobin available to tissues. The half-life of CO in room air is about 5 h. The treatment of choice is 100% O_2, which reduces the half-life to 1 h. Hyperbaric O_2 can speed this process but is not necessary.

210.   The answer is E (all). (Miller, 4/e. pp 2431–2432.) Carbon monoxide poisoning is the most common cause of death in people involved in fires. One must have a high index of suspicion for CO poisoning. Treatment is with 100% oxygen or hyperbaric oxygen if available. An arterial blood gas will also give a carboxyhemoglobin level that will be helpful with the diagnosis. Patients with severe CO poisoning do not hyperventilate in response to metabolic acidosis. CO diffuses into cells, binding to myoglobin and cytochromes. This may be why measured levels of COHb do not always correlate with the severity of the clinical presentation.

211.   The answer is C (2, 4). (Miller, 4/e. p 1084.) Succinylcholine and halothane are agents that are known to trigger malignant hyperthermia. All the other inhalational agents have been associated with malignant hyperthermia as well. Lidocaine and atropine do not trigger the syndrome.

212.   The answer is A (1, 2, 3). (Miller, 4/e. pp 1085–1086.) An increased susceptibility to malignant hyperthermia has been documented for Duchenne muscular dystrophy and occasionally reported with occult myopathies and central core disease. No association with cerebral palsy has been demonstrated.

213.   The answer is C (2, 4). (Barash, 3/e. pp 492–494, 496–498.) Patients who have MH-susceptible relatives and have an elevated CPK are at high risk for the disease, but a normal CPK does not rule out susceptibility. The only known unsafe anesthetic drugs are the potent inhalational agents and depolarizing muscle relaxants, such as succinylcholine and decamethonium. Avoidance of a triggering technique is highly effective in preventing an MH response, and so dantrolene need not be given to every MH-susceptible patient (this is controversial) since it can cause muscle weakness and other side effects. It is as effective in treating as in preventing an MH response.

214.   The answer is A (1, 2, 3). (Stoelting, *Pharmacology,* 2/e. pp 546–547.) Dantrolene's site of action is not entirely understood, but the drug seems to inhibit the release of calcium from the sarcoplasmic reticulum. It also may speed reuptake of calcium into the sarcoplasmic reticulum. The drug has no effect on neuromuscular transmission. Dantrolene is dissolved in sterile water: 50 mL of water to 20 mg of dantrolene.

215.   The answer is E (all). (Stoelting, *Pharmacology,* 2/e. pp 360–361, 546–547.) Skeletal muscle weakness is the most common side effect and may interfere with ventilation. The incidence of hepatitis is approximately 0.5 percent in patients treated for more than 60 days.

216.   The answer is D (4). (Stoelting, *Anesthesia and Co-Existing Disease,* 3/e. pp 524–525.) The cause of NMS is not known, and its incidence is not associated with MH triggering agents. The hyperthermia, hypertonicity of skeletal muscle, and cardiovascular manifestations are treated symptomatically. Dantrolene is useful in treating the hypertonicity of skeletal muscle.

217. The answer is D (4). (Barash, 3/e. pp 1188–1190, 1196.) Fluid needs are great, but the recommended amount is 2 to 4 mL/kg per hour for each percent of body burned. Follow vital signs and urine output as final monitors. Evaporative losses, high metabolism, and exposure tend to lead to hypothermia in burn patients. Burn patients receiving succinyl-choline can have an abnormally high release of potassium, leading to cardiac arrest. Resistance to nondepolarizing muscle relaxants is due to the proliferation of extrajunctional receptors, which are less responsive to these drugs. These patients have severe pain and require high doses of narcotics.

218. The answer is D (4). (Stoelting, *Anesthesia and Co-Existing Disease,* 3/e. pp 624–625.) The greatest risk for a massive hyperkalemic response appears to be 10 to 30 days after a burn. There is a change in the sensitivity to nondepolarizing muscle relaxants, with marked resistance to these drugs. Plasma albumin fraction is down, while alpha$_1$ acid glycoprotein is increased. Inhaled anesthestics work very well in this population, as does ketamine.

219. The answer is A (1, 2, 3). (Stoelting, *Pharmacology,* 2/e. pp 373–378.) Care should be taken to avoid additive effects of tricyclic antidepressants and anticholinergics. Tricyclic antidepressants block the centrally mediated antihypertensive effects of clonidine, presumably by displacing norepinephrine. Tricyclic antidepressants increase the requirements for inhalational anesthetics. This is theoretically due to increased levels of norepinephrine. The exaggerated response can be seen with the use of indirect-acting sympathomimetics because of increased circulating catecholamines.

220. The answer is D (4). (Miller, 4/e. p 992.) Phenothiazines have dopamine-receptor blocking properties, which may interfere with the action of dopamine. They also have significant alpha blocking properties, which may cause orthostatic hypotension. Patients on phenothiazines are highly sensitive to narcotics, barbiturates, and CNS depressing drugs. Seizure threshold is lowered in these patients.

221. The answer is E (all). (Stoelting, *Pharmacology,* 2/e. pp 378–381.) MAO inhibitors inhibit enzyme activity in the liver. Orthostatic hypotension may be due to the accumulation of octopamine, a false neurotransmitter, in the nerve endings. All opioids, but specifically meperidine, may lead to hyperthermia when used in the presence of MAO inhibitors.

222. The answer is C (2, 4). (Miller, 4/e. pp 562–563, 991–992.) Though meperidine has the most severe interaction with MAO inhibitors, most of the narcotics have been reported in untoward incidents with MAO inhibitors. Because MAO inhibitors cause a buildup of intracellular norepinephrine, indirect-acting sympathetic drugs can release large amounts of this neurotransmitter into the circulation and cause exaggerated sympathetic responses. Direct-acting sympathomimetic drugs can also cause an exaggerated response, but this is due to a denervation hypersensitivity or up-regulation of adrenergic receptors. Regional block using local anesthetics is probably safe for pain control.

223.   The answer is A (1, 2, 3). (Stoelting, *Pharmacology,* 2/e. pp 371–373.) Up to 95 percent of lithium is eliminated by the kidneys. In addition to furosemide, thiazide diuretics can increase lithium levels to the toxic range. Lithium causes sedation in patients, potentially decreasing their anesthetic requirement.

224.   The answer is E (all). (Barash, 3/e. pp 1319–1322, 1327.) TENS probably activates large afferent fibers, which then stimulate inhibitory dorsal horn neurons to prevent nociceptive transmission. It is possible that endogenous opioids are also released. Local anesthetics block sensory, motor, and sympathetic neuronal transmission. PCA maintains a steady-state drug level in patients. It prevents the emergence of pain and gives patients a sense of control over their condition, which eliminates some anxiety. Intrathecal narcotics do modulate supraspinal opioid receptor sites, but they also suppress nociceptive reception in the spinal cord.

225.   The answer is A (1, 2, 3). (Miller, 4/e. pp 2359–2361.) Neurolytic blocks should be considered only in patients with short life expectancy who are suffering from pain of malignancies. Most of these blocks are applied in the subarachnoid space because of the incidence of denervation dysesthetic pain after peripheral block. Because the neurolytic agents destroy all tissue with which they come in contact, it is critical that diagnostic blocks with local anesthetics be done first. This assures that the block will actually take away the pain and helps increase the accuracy of placement.

226.   The answer is D (4). (Barash, 3/e. p 1351.) Causalgia is a form of reflex sympathetic dystrophy associated with injury to major nerve trunks and often is due to gunshot wounds. Pain usually starts at the site of injury, can spread to other areas, and can be exacerbated by stimulation of the sympathetic nervous system, such as bright lights, loud noises, and anxiety. Treatment by peripheral nerve blockade is useless. Early blockade of the major sympathetic ganglion that serves the area of injury seems to be most effective.

227.   The answer is A (1, 2, 3). (Barash, 3/e. pp 1349–1351.) RSD is a pain syndrome that includes autonomic dysfunction and dystrophic changes and usually occurs after trauma or surgery. Autonomic changes also include cyanosis and episodes of severe vasoconstriction. Hyperalgesia is common; patients complain of extreme pain on light touch and pain beyond the site of injury.

228.   The answer is D (4). (Miller, 4/e. p 2350.) Central pain states are thought to arise from within the CNS, not peripherally. Therefore, none of the traditional forms of analgesics or sedatives afford much relief. A combination of phenytoin and carbamazepine often works well for central pain of a spasmatic or episodic nature, such as tic douloureux (trigeminal neuralgia). Phantom limb pain can be resistant to treatment, although calcitonin and combinations of antidepressants and fluphenazine have been effective in some patients.

229. **The answer is A (1, 2, 3).** (Stoelting, *Pharmacology,* 2/e. pp 282–283.) Toxicity in neonates is a possibility with aminophylline. Halothane more than isoflurane or enflurane may be associated with dysrhythmias. Metabolism of aminophylline is increased in cigarette smokers.

230. **The answer is C (2, 4).** (Miller, 4/e. pp 992–993.) Beta$_2$ selective drugs, such as terbutaline, in high doses stimulate beta$_1$ receptors. Thus, halothane-induced dysrhythmias can occur in their presence. Aminophylline causes the release of norepinephrine and prevents its breakdown by inhibiting phosphodiesterase. Steroids have no effect on myocardial irritability.

231. **The answer is B (1, 3).** (Barash, 3/e. p 982.) Metoclopramide and succinylcholine increase LES tone. Succinylcholine also increases intragastric pressure. Atropine, scopolamine, and glycopyrrolate reduce LES tone, as do thiopental, opioids, and inhaled anesthetics.

232. **The answer is B (1, 3).** (Stoelting, *Anesthesia and Co-Existing Disease,* 3/e. pp 283–284.) Carcinoid tumors release vasoactive substances, such as serotonin, which trigger bronchoconstriction, chronic abdominal pain, hyperglycemia, and cardiac dysrhythmias, among other problems. Histamine-releasing drugs and catecholamines such as epinephrine may cause an exacerbation of symptoms. The growth hormone somatostatin inhibits release of vasoactive substances from carcinoid tumors. Carcinoid tumors are quite common, but only 5 percent of patients who have tumors actually develop the syndrome.

CARDIOVASCULAR SYSTEM

Directions: Each question below contains five suggested responses. Select the **one best** response to each question.

233. All the following may alter stimulation thresholds for pacemakers EXCEPT

(A) hypokalemia
(B) hyperkalemia
(C) hypoxemia
(D) isoflurane
(E) catecholamines

234. The definition of bipolar pacing in cardiac pacemakers is as follows:

(A) The pacemaker will have both an epicardial electrode and an endocardial electrode as backup in case one or the other fails

(B) The pacemaker will have one electrode in the atrium and one electrode in the ventricle to provide atrioventricular sequential pacing

(C) The pacemaker will have the placement of both the stimulating (negative) electrode and the ground (positive) electrode in the cardiac chamber that is being paced

(D) The pacemaker will have the stimulating electrode in the cardiac chamber that is being paced and the ground electrode distal from this chamber

(E) The pacemaker will have the stimulating electrode distal from the heart and the ground electrode in the chamber that is being paced

235. The first three letters of generic coding for the identification of pacemakers can be defined as follows:

(A)   First letter, programmable functions of pacemaker; second letter, cardiac chamber in which electrical activity is sensed; third letter, response of generator to sensed R and P waves

(B)   First letter, cardiac chamber in which electrical activity is sensed; second letter, cardiac chamber paced; third letter, response of generator to sinus R and P waves

(C)   First letter, cardiac chamber paced; second letter, cardiac chamber in which electrical activity is sensed; third letter, response of generator to sensed R and P waves

(D)   First letter, response of generator to sensed R and P waves; second letter, cardiac chamber in which electrical activity is sensed; third letter, cardiac chamber paced

(E)   First letter, antitachycardia function of pacemaker; second letter, cardiac chamber paced; third letter, cardiac chamber in which electrical activity is sensed

236. The most common cause of temporary pacemaker malfunction is interruption of contact between the electrode wire and the endocardium. This may be caused by all the following EXCEPT

(A)   electrocautery
(B)   exercise
(C)   blunt trauma
(D)   cardioversion
(E)   positive pressure ventilation

237. Concerning pacemakers, hysteresis may be defined as

(A)   the energy source (battery) and electrical circuitry necessary for pacing

(B)   the difference between the heart rate at which pacing begins and the pacing rate

(C)   the anatomic placement of the pulse generator relative to the skin

(D)   how the pacemaker will respond when an R wave or P wave is sensed

(E)   the menu of programmable functions the pacemaker can perform

238. All the following are true concerning electrocautery and pacemakers EXCEPT

(A)   the anesthesiologist should know how to convert the pacemaker to the asynchronous mode, i.e., fixed rate, with either a magnet or a reprogramming device

(B)   the electrocautery dispersion plate should be placed as far away from the pulse generator as possible

(C)   a magnet should be put on the pulse generator prophylactically before any electrocautery begins

(D)   if at all possible, bipolar cautery should be used

(E)   blood flow should be monitored in a way not affected by electocautery

239. Referring to the diagram of the ventricular pressure-volume loop below, stroke volume is equal to the volume at

(A) point A plus point B
(B) point B plus point C
(C) point B minus point C
(D) point B minus point D
(E) point D plus point A

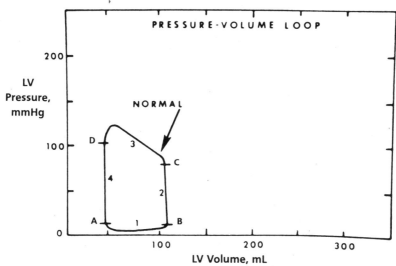

From Jackson JM, Thomas SJ, Lowenstein E: *Seminars in Anesthesia*, 1982, with permission.

240. In a patient with aortic stenosis,

(A) aortic regurgitation is a rare associated finding
(B) high left ventricular systolic pressures are characteristic
(C) a transvalvular gradient of 25 mmHg usually is associated with hemodynamic instability
(D) a valve area of 3.5 cm² would be expected to be associated with severe obstruction to flow
(E) the major compensatory mechanism of the left ventricle is dilation

241. All the following statements regarding aortic stenosis are true EXCEPT

(A) the incidence of sudden death is increased in patients with aortic stenosis
(B) angina, dyspnea on exertion, and syncopy is a classic triad of symptoms
(C) goals of anesthetic management include maintenance of normal sinus rhythm, avoidance of tachycardia, and avoidance of large reductions in systemic vascular resistance
(D) angina may occur in the absence of coronary artery disease
(E) aortic stenosis is characterized by a diastolic murmur

242. All the following statements are true EXCEPT

 (A) pericardial fluid volume is normally 20 to 25 mL
 (B) cardiac tamponade is characterized by a decrease in stroke volume (SV) and blood pressure (BP)
 (C) pulsus paradoxus is a sign of cardiac tamponade
 (D) pulmonary capillary wedge pressure (PCWP) is normally elevated relative to right atrial pressure (RAP) and right ventricular pressure (RVP) in cardiac tamponade
 (E) increased intrathoracic pressure, as seen with positive pressure ventilation (PPV), can be hazardous in the presence of cardiac tamponade

243. The risk factor most commonly associated with descending aortic dissection is

 (A) atherosclerosis
 (B) end-stage syphilis
 (C) blunt chest trauma
 (D) hypertension
 (E) Marfan's syndrome

244. A rare postoperative complication that can occur after abdominal aortic aneurysmectomy is

 (A) renal failure
 (B) pulmonary failure
 (C) spinal cord infarction
 (D) hypovolemia
 (E) myocardial dysfunction

245. The major cause of morbidity and mortality after surgery on the aorta and its major branches is

 (A) perioperative myocardial ischemia and infarction
 (B) acute renal failure
 (C) graft sepsis
 (D) spinal cord infarction
 (E) pulmonary failure

246. Aortic cross-clamping may produce myocardial ischemic changes that will most often be detected in which monitored ECG lead?

 (A) II
 (B) AVL
 (C) V_1
 (D) AVF
 (E) V_5

247. The most sensitive monitor for myocardial ischemia in a patient undergoing major vascular surgery is

 (A) continuous monitoring of mixed venous oxygen saturation (SVO_2)
 (B) thermodilution cardiac outputs
 (C) wall-motion abnormalities of the left ventricle delineated by intraoperative two-dimensional transesophageal echocardiography
 (D) ST segment changes of ECG lead V_5
 (E) changes in calculated systemic vascular resistance

248. All the following may cause a decrease in renal cortical perfusion after aortic cross-clamping EXCEPT

(A) increase in the secretion of renin-angiotensin
(B) increase in the blood level of catecholamines
(C) decrease in cardiac output
(D) embolization of atheromatous material to the kidney
(E) decrease in renal vascular resistance

249. Methods of renal protection before aortic cross-clamping may include all the following EXCEPT

(A) intravenous mannitol 0.25 to 1.0 g/kg
(B) intravenous furosemide 5 to 50 mg
(C) infusion of low-dose dopamine 1 to 3 μg/kg/min
(D) epidural anesthesia with a sympathetic blockade level to T6
(E) systemic and renal artery calcium channel blockade

250. The complications that occur secondary to acute dissection of the thoracic aorta (ascending and descending) may include all the following EXCEPT

(A) acute aortic insufficiency
(B) acute pericardial tamponade
(C) compromise of circulation to the brain and heart
(D) acute aortic stenosis
(E) compromise of circulation to the spinal cord and subdiaphragmatic viscera

251. The major goal of premedication in a patient before surgery for abdominal aortic aneurysm is to

(A) provide amnesia
(B) prevent postoperative nausea and vomiting
(C) decrease the risk of aspiration
(D) provide a relaxed and tranquil patient
(E) smooth the onset of anesthesia

252. Hypotension during or after carotid artery surgery may be caused by

(A) stroke after carotid endarterectomy
(B) intraoperative denervation of the carotid sinus
(C) intraoperative denervation of the carotid body
(D) plaque removal from the region of the carotid baroreceptors
(E) intraoperative transection of the recurrent laryngeal nerve

253. A possible cause of hypertension after carotid endarterectomy is

(A) trauma to the recurrent laryngeal nerve
(B) plaque removal from the carotid baroreceptor
(C) transection of the phrenic nerve
(D) trauma to the stellate ganglion
(E) denervation of the carotid sinus

Directions: Each question below contains four suggested responses of which **one or more** is correct. Select

(A)	if	**1, 2, and 3**	are correct
(B)	if	**1 and 3**	are correct
(C)	if	**2 and 4**	are correct
(D)	if	**4**	is correct
(E)	if	**1, 2, 3, and 4**	are correct

254. Direct cardiac massage may be more efficacious than closed cardiac massage

  (1) because resuscitation can be successful long after the onset of arrest
  (2) and probably should be used more often in routine cardiac arrest
  (3) because there is improved outcome even after closed chest massage has gone on for 20 min or more
  (4) in patients with penetrating chest trauma

255. Bradyarrhythmias can be

  (1) caused by stimulation of the carotid sinus
  (2) seen with high sympathetic blockade
  (3) brought on by drugs such as narcotics
  (4) caused by pressure on the eyes

256. Bradycardias should be treated

  (1) if the heart rate falls below 45 beats per minute
  (2) if there are signs of poor peripheral perfusion
  (3) initially with calcium channel blockers
  (4) if there are sustained and multifocal ectopic ventricular beats

257. True statements about dysrhythmias and their treatment include which of the following?

  (1) The treatment of choice for complete heart block with a slow idioventricular escape rhythm at 15 to 30 beats per minute is atropine followed by an isoproterenol infusion titrated to a heart rate consistent with an adequate blood pressure
  (2) Sodium bicarbonate is no longer a first-line drug in the treatment of electromechanical dissociation unless hyperkalemia is present
  (3) If atrial fibrillation or flutter is accompanied by a rapid ventricular response, synchronized cardioversion should not exceed 75 joule because of the risk of converting to ventricular fibrillation
  (4) Drugs that affect heart rate and rhythm and that can be given effectively and safely via the endotracheal tube include lidocaine, atropine, and epinephrine

258. Sinus tachyarrhythmias seen in the operating room may be due to

  (1) hypovolemia
  (2) hypercarbia
  (3) hypoxia
  (4) heart failure

259. Atrial flutter and atrial fibrillation

    (1)   are rarely seen with preexisting heart disease
    (2)   may be signs of pulmonary embolism
    (3)   are rarely of significance and can be observed
    (4)   may be signs of hyperthyroidism

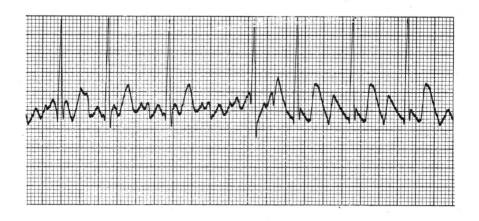

260. Premature ventricular contractions (PVCs) are often seen in the operating room (15 percent of all arrhythmias). True statements regarding PVCs include

    (1)   they rarely indicate anything other than ischemia
    (2)   they are more common in patients with preexisting coronary disease
    (3)   they are easily differentiated from premature atrial contractions
    (4)   new onset of this dysrhythmia should always be investigated as to its cause

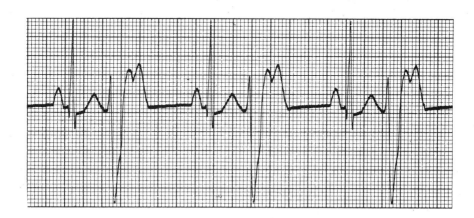

SUMMARY OF DIRECTIONS

A	B	C	D	E
1,2,3	1,3	2,4	4	All are
only	only	only	only	correct

261. True statements regarding ventricular tachycardia, which is potentially life-threatening, include which of the following?

(1) In a stable patient (no hypotension, unconsciousness, or signs of ischemia), atropine 0.5 mg is the initial treatment of choice

(2) If the patient is pulseless, the ventricular fibrillation protocol should be instituted immediately

(3) Cardioversion, starting at 300 joule, should be instituted in a patient with a systolic blood pressure of 70 and 2-mm ST depressions on the ECG

(4) After successful treatment, an antiarrhythmic drug should be infused to maintain suppression of the ectopic focus

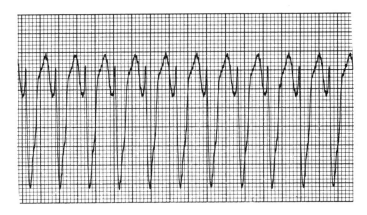

262. Pulseless electrical activity (PEA) can have a variety of etiologies. True statements include

(1) PEA is pulseless, with no effective cardiac output, and CPR should be initiated

(2) massive acute thromboembolism is not a cause of PEA

(3) electrical cardioversion is of little use in treatment

(4) atropine is the agent most useful in treatment

263. True statements concerning phenytoin include

(1) antidysrhythmic action is due to an initial release of catecholamines

(2) phenytoin effectively prolongs the Q-T interval on ECG

(3) phenytoin is an effective treatment for ventricular fibrillation refractory to other therapies

(4) phenytoin is the drug of choice for dysrhythmias induced by digitalis toxicity

264. Ventricular fibrillation is a life-threatening rhythm. True statements include

(1) it usually is associated with a weak pulse
(2) fine ventricular fibrillation is easier to convert than coarse ventricular fibrillation
(3) the pattern on the ECG usually is regular and smooth
(4) immediate electrical defibrillation is the treatment of choice

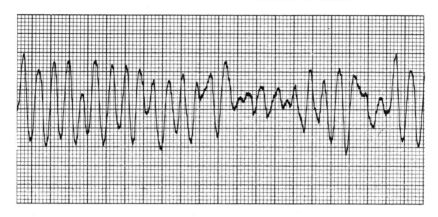

265. During a Valsalva maneuver,

(1) venous pressures of the head and upper extremities increase
(2) venous return to the right side of the heart decreases
(3) cardiac output and blood pressure both decrease
(4) a reflex increase in heart rate usually occurs

266. With regard to the coronary circulation,

(1) it constitutes approximately 5 percent of the cardiac output
(2) the most important regulators of coronary vascular tone are local metabolic factors
(3) more than 80 percent of coronary perfusion occurs during diastole
(4) autoregulation of coronary perfusion occurs between perfusion pressures of 50 and 120 mmHg

267. True statements about the systemic circulation include which of the following?

(1) Tracing the circulation from the aorta to the venae cavae, the largest drop in blood pressure occurs at the arterioles
(2) The incisura, or dicrotic notch, in an arterial pressure tracing from the aorta represents the end of systole
(3) When an arterial transducer affixed to an IV pole 10 cm from the floor has a zero reference point at the right atrium, which is 50 cm from the floor, the transducer suddenly falls to the floor; the systolic pressure will read 7 mmHg higher than it did before the transducer fell
(4) Pulse pressure is lower in a peripheral artery (e.g., dorsalis pedis) than in a central artery (e.g., aorta)

SUMMARY OF DIRECTIONS

A	B	C	D	E
1,2,3 only	1,3 only	2,4 only	4 only	All are correct

268. True statements about cardiac physiology include

 (1) coronary perfusion on both the right side and the left side of the heart occurs only during diastole
 (2) tachycardia and increased ventricular size will decrease coronary flow reserve
 (3) coronary arteries maintain a constant blood flow between perfusion pressures of 40 to 50 mmHg
 (4) adenosine is the most important mediator of coronary vascular tone

269. Nifedipine is a calcium channel blocker that

 (1) is both a cardiac depressant and a vasodilator
 (2) is indicated for coronary vasospasm
 (3) can cause a reflex tachycardia
 (4) is available for intravenous and sublingual administration

270. Cyclosporine, which inhibits T-cell function,

 (1) is toxic to marrow
 (2) is potentially nephrotoxic
 (3) often leads to mild hypotension
 (4) promotes hyperplasia of gingiva

271. Inadequate heparinization on bypass may present as

 (1) fibrin accumulation on the walls of the bypass reservoir
 (2) thickening of blood in the pericardium
 (3) coagulopathic bleeding
 (4) ACT greater than 400 s

272. True statements about bypass surgery include which of the following?

 (1) Malpositioning of the aortic cannula from aortic dissection, inadequate size of the aortic cannula, and occlusion of the aortic line can lead to high aortic line pressure
 (2) Aortic dissection may result in both a decrease in venous return and an elevated aortic line pressure
 (3) The remedy for a low venous saturation on bypass includes improvement of possibly inadequate perfusion by increasing flow or increasing the depth of anesthesia and providing muscle relaxation to overcome the increase in oxygen demand
 (4) Failure in the oxygenator would manifest as a decrease in arterial saturation and an increase in arterial CO_2

273. Which of the following congenital cardiac lesions may require the placement of a Blalock-Taussig shunt?

 (1) Tetralogy of Fallot
 (2) Atrioventricular canal
 (3) Pulmonary atresia
 (4) Ebstein's anomaly

274. Which of the following may cause low venous return during cardiopulmonary bypass?

(1) Air in the tubing between the vena cava and the venous return reservoir
(2) Aortic dissection
(3) Occult bleeding
(4) Vena cava too high compared with the venous return reservoir

275. Regarding patients with regurgitant valvular lesions,

(1) in mitral regurgitation, the amount of regurgitant flow correlates with the size of the *v* wave seen in the pulmonary capillary wedge pressure tracing
(2) in mitral or aortic regurgitation, maintenance of low systemic vascular resistance is desirable
(3) in mitral or aortic regurgitation, maintenance of mild tachycardia is desirable
(4) in aortic regurgitation, PA catheters may be helpful in determining the response to peripheral dilating drugs

276. True statements regarding mitral stenosis include

(1) maneuvers that increase pulmonary vascular resistance are beneficial because they augment preload and therefore cardiac output
(2) tachycardia is expected to be more detrimental than bradycardia
(3) LV dysfunction is commonly seen in pure stenotic lesions
(4) pulmonary capillary wedge pressure will overestimate left ventricular end-diastolic pressure

277. True statements about tricuspid regurgitation include

(1) it is rarely associated with pulmonary hypertension
(2) it is commonly associated with infectious endocarditis from IV drug abuse
(3) anesthetic management includes fluid restriction
(4) nitrous oxide may increase the regurgitant fraction

278. Side effects of protamine administration include

(1) anaphylactic or anaphylactoid reactions
(2) hypotension secondary to histamine release
(3) pulmonary hypertension
(4) ventricular arrhythmias

279. Side effects associated with heparin therapy include

(1) altered protein binding of propranolol
(2) allergic reactions
(3) hypotension after infusion of high doses
(4) thrombocytopenia from platelet aggregation

280. Management of patients with heparin resistance secondary to antithrombin III deficiency who will undergo cardiopulmonary bypass includes

(1) pretreating for several days with warfarin (Coumadin)
(2) making the initial heparin dose 600 units/kg
(3) hydrocortisone 100 mg IV before the operation
(4) transfusion of fresh frozen plasma (FFP)

SUMMARY OF DIRECTIONS

A	B	C	D	E
1,2,3	1,3	2,4	4	All are
only	only	only	only	correct

281. In the ventricular pressure-volume loop shown below,

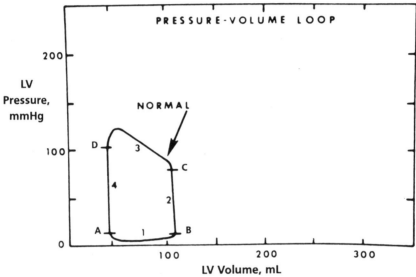

From Jackson JM, Thomas SJ, Lowenstein E: *Seminars in Anesthesia*, 1982, with permission.

    (1)   A represents mitral valve opening
    (2)   B represents mitral value closure
    (3)   C represents aortic valve opening
    (4)   D represents end-systolic volume

282. With regard to pacemakers and electrocautery,

(1) the electrocautery "ground plate" should be placed as close as possible to the pulse generator

(2) the electrocautery current should be kept as low as possible

(3) long, widely paced bursts minimize the chance of pacemaker malfunction

(4) myopotentials as a result of fasciculations after succinylcholine administration may cause pacemaker malfunction

283. In evaluating pacemaker function preoperatively,

(1) reason for placement of the pacemaker, date of placement, and type of pulse generator are all necessary information

(2) a regular peripheral pulse of 70 to 72 beats per minute is compatible with the presence of a VOO pacemaker

(3) a regular peripheral pulse of 70 to 72 beats per minute is compatible with the presence of a VVI pacemaker

(4) a chest x-ray is helpful

284. True statements regarding noninvasive transcutaneous pacers (NTPs) include

(1) they are better at improving the outcome of bradysystolic arrests than are transvenous pacers

(2) the leads should be placed over areas of minimal muscle mass

(3) they deliver low-density constant-current impulses

(4) hemodynamic response is similar to that with transvenous pacers

285. Regarding artificial cardiac pacemakers,

(1) a pacemaker designated VOO is also known as a *demand* pacemaker

(2) a pacemaker designated VVI is also known as an *asynchronous* pacemaker

(3) a DVI designation on a pacemaker means that it senses both the atrium and the ventricle but paces only the ventricle, while the pulse generation responds to a sensed R or P wave in an inhibitory fashion

(4) a DDD pacemaker may increase cardiac output 30 percent over a VVI pacemaker

CARDIOVASCULAR SYSTEM

233. **The answer is D.** (Stoelting, *Anesthesia and Co-Existing Disease,* 3/e. p 66.) Hypokalemia results in an increased stimulation threshold, and hyperkalemia results in a decreased stimulation threshold. Halothane isoflurane, and enflurane have never been implicated in changing the stimulation threshold.

234. **The answer is C.** (Stoelting, *Anesthesia and Co-Existing Disease,* 3/e. p 63.) Bipolar pacing is defined as having both the stimulating (negative) electrode and the ground (positive) electrode in the chamber that is being paced. Unipolar pacing is defined as having the negative electrode in the chamber that is being paced and the positive electrode at some point distant from the chamber. Bipolar pacemakers are less susceptible to interference, such as electrocautery, because the negative and positive electrodes are close together.

235. **The answer is C.** (Stoelting, *Anesthesia and Co-Existing Disease,* 3/e. p 64.) The three-letter generic code for identification of a pacemaker can be defined as follows: First letter, cardiac chamber paced; second letter, cardiac chamber in which electrical activity is sensed; third letter, response of generator to sensed R and P waves. Therefore, a VVI pacemaker may be defined as follows: (1) the ventricle is paced, (2) sensing occurs in the ventricle, and (3) the response to a sensed R wave is that the pacemaker will be inhibited.

236. **The answer is A.** (Miller, 4/e. p 957.) When temporary transvenous pacemakers are used, the most common cause of malfunction is disconnection of the stimulating electrode from the myocardium. What one will see on the ECG is continuous pacing spikes without capture. On physical examination, no pulse will be detected, and there will be no evidence of blood flow if pulse oximetry or an arterial line is present. Treatment consists of advancing the stimulating electrode forward until there is capture. If this fails, an external pacer can be used or pharmacologic measures with atropine or isoproterenol can be attempted. Causes of electrode disconnection include exercise, blunt trauma, cardioversion, positive pressure ventilation, and central line placement but not electrocautery.

237. **The answer is B.** (Stoelting, *Anesthesia and Co-Existing Disease,* 3/e. p 63.) Hysteresis is defined as the difference between the heart rate at which pacing begins and the pacing rate. A change in hysteresis can signal any or all of the following: battery failure, lead fracture, and reprogramming of the pacemaker.

238. **The answer is C.** (Miller, 4/e. p 957.) Before putting a magnet on a pulse generator, the anesthesiologist should be aware of what the magnet may do to the pacemaker. Some pacemakers will be converted to the asynchronous mode when a magnet is placed, while others may be reprogrammed. This may be dangerous to the patient. Bipolar electrocautery will not interfere with pacemaker function.

239. **The answer is D.** (Barash, 2/e. pp 1007–1008.) Stroke volume is defined as the difference between end-diastolic volume (EDV) and end-systolic volume (ESV). Since points B and D represent EDV and ESV, respectively, stroke volume is the difference between the volumes at these points.

240. **The answer is B.** (Stoelting, *Anesthesia and Co-Existing Disease,* 3/e. pp 31–32.) High LV systolic pressures are characteristic of aortic stenosis. The normal aortic valve area is 2.6 to 3.5 cm^2. The major compensatory mechanism of the left ventricle in aortic stenosis is concentric hypertrophy. Aortic regurgitation is a common concurrent finding, and transvalvular gradients greater than 50 mmHg are usually hemodynamically significant.

241. **The answer is E.** (Stoelting, *Anesthesia and Co-Existing Disease,* 3/e. pp 31–32.) The characteristic murmur of aortic stenosis is systolic, not diastolic. It is best heard in the second right interspace and often radiates to the carotids.

242. **The answer is D.** (Stoelting, *Anesthesia and Co-Existing Disease,* 3/e. pp 107–112.) Classically, the "equalization of pressures" seen in cardiac tamponade refers to the equalization of RAP, RVP, and PCWP. Other signs include distant heart sounds and sympathetic stimulation.

243. **The answer is D.** (Miller, 4/e. pp 1884–1885.) Hypertensive vascular disease is present in 70 to 90 percent of patients who develop acute dissection of the descending thoracic aorta and is the most common cause. Connective tissue diseases, infection, atherosclerosis, and blunt chest trauma less commonly cause this problem.

244. **The answer is C.** (Miller, 4/e. p 1879.) Spinal cord infarction occurs with a frequency of approximately 1 in 1000 after abdominal aortic aneurysmectomy. One possible reason is that the artery of Adamkiewicz arises from the aorta in a highly anomalous fashion and may arise infrarenally. Even monitoring of somatosensory evoked potentials may not be adequate to assess this problem, because only the posterior portion of the spinal cord is monitored.

245. **The answer is A.** (Miller, 4/e. p 1870.) The leading cause of death after major vascular surgery is myocardial ischemia and infarction. The great majority of patients who present for major vascular surgery have underlying severe, diffuse atherosclerosis that affects multiple organ systems. More than 50 percent of these patients manifest signs of ischemic heart disease preoperatively. Of the perioperative deaths in patients who have undergone major vascular surgery, 40 to 60 percent can be attributed to cardiac dysfunction. This is three to four times higher than any other cause of death.

246. **The answer is E.** (Miller, 4/e. p 1872.) Aortic cross-clamping increases impedance to left ventricular work. As a result, there can be an increase in myocardial oxygen demand, which may then outstrip supply. This may lead to myocardial ischemia. ST segment depressions usually signify endocardial ischemia, while ST segment elevations (although less common) may signify transmural ischemia. If the ECG is used as a monitor of ischemia, 75 to 85 percent of ischemic changes will occur along the V_5 lead. The V_5 monitors the distribution of blood flow of the left main and left anterior descending (LAD) coronary arteries, which supply blood to the septum and the majority of the left ventricle

247. **The answer is C.** (Miller, 4/e. p 1872.) There is considerable interest in the use of two-dimensional transesophageal echocardiography (2-D TEE) intraoperatively for the detection of ischemia. It is believed that the mere occurrence of left ventricular and septal wall–motion abnormalities is indicative of a new onset of ischemia. The occurrence of these wall-motion abnormalities may precede changes such as increases in filling pressures, onset of v waves, decreases in cardiac index, and decreases in SVO_2 that are indicators of ischemia when one is using pulmonary artery catheter monitoring. Wall–motion abnormalities also precede signs of ischemia on ECG. There is strong evidence that 2-D TEE monitoring may be more sensitive than pulmonary artery monitoring or ECG monitoring for ischemia.

248. **The answer is E.** (Miller, 4/e. pp 1878–1879.) Abdominal aortic cross-clamping has significant effects on renal perfusion and function. Cortical blood flow is decreased. This may be caused by increases in hormones such as renin-angiotensin, catecholamines, ADH, aldosterone, and corticosteroids. There is an increase in renal vascular resistance. Decreases in cardiac output—by decreases in filling pressures, decreases in contractility, or increases in systemic vascular resistance—also may decrease renal cortical perfusion. Surgical manipulations of the kidneys and embolization of atheromatous material to the kidney also have been implicated in decreasing renal blood flow.

249. **The answer is D.** (Miller, 4/e. pp 1878–1879.) Epidural anesthesia with resultant sympathectomy to level T6 does not increase renal blood flow. Mannitol causes renal vasodilation and may have a direct effect of increasing cortical blood flow. The net effect of mannitol is to improve renal blood flow. Some studies have indicated that mannitol used before cross-clamping may prevent acute renal failure. Dopamine 1 to 3 μg/kg/min improves renal cortical blood flow via dopaminergic stimulation. Furosemide improves urine output, which some sources feel is protective. Maintenance of cardiac output ensures normal renal perfusion. These maneuvers to prevent postoperative acute renal failure are worthwhile because of the high mortality associated with renal failure. Systemic calcium channel blockade with nicardipine and direct administration of verapamil into the renal arteries may prevent renal artery constriction.

250. **The answer is D.** (Miller, 4/e. pp 1884–1886.) An acute dissection of the thoracic aorta is a catastrophic event. Initially, there is a tear in the intima of the aorta. Blood forces its way through this tear and then creates a longitudinal tear that will progress both proximally and distally. Dissections are classified according to where the initial intimal tear occurred. Proximal dissection can cause acute aortic insufficiency and acute pericardial tamponade. Dissection also can occlude the coronary ostia and thereby occlude coronary artery blood flow. There also may be interruption of blood flow to the brain, spinal cord, and viscera. Acute aortic stenosis is not a complication.

251. **The answer is D.** (Miller, 4/e. p 1871.) Although all the listed choices are often the goals of premedication, the primary goal for any major vascular surgery is to provide a relaxed and tranquil patient. These patients often have underlying diffuse atherosclerotic disease. The tachycardia and hypertension often seen in anxious patients may precipitate myocardial ischemia, dysrhythmias, or, in the case of an aneurysm, rupture.

252. **The answer is D.** (Miller, 4/e. p 1869.) After hypovolemia, cardiac dysfunction, hypoxia, and hypercarbia have been ruled out, hypotension with bradycardia may be due to plaque removal from the carotid baroreceptors. It is believed that when significant amounts of plaque have been removed from the baroreceptors, there is increased neural discharge to the CNS because of this perceived increase in blood pressure. Reflexly, the central nervous system increases vagal tone and parasympathetic nervous system discharge, which results in hypotension and bradycardia. Judicious use of vasopressors may be necessary. This problem usually abates within 12 to 24 h with readjustment to the new homeostasis.

253. **The answer is E.** (Miller, 4/e. p 1869.) Postoperative hypertension after carotid artery surgery is extremely common. The differential diagnosis includes all the following: poorly controlled primary hypertension, hypoxia, hypercarbia, pain, a full bladder, and airway compromise. Another cause of hypertension is denervation of the carotid sinus baroreceptor during intraoperative mobilization of the carotid bifurcations. This leads to loss of baroreceptor function. Judicious use of short-acting antihypertensives such as esmolol, sodium nitroprusside, and labetalol is helpful until baroreceptor function has returned.

254. **The answer is D (4).** (American Heart Association 1994 Textbook. pp 11.3–11.4.) Though open cardiac massage can be successful, it is so only if started within 15 min of the onset of cardiac arrest. It has not been shown to work after closed chest compressions have gone on for some time, nor should it be used in routine arrests. However, with penetrating chest trauma, open chest massage allows for better evaluation and treatment of possible tamponade and great vessel injury. It also may be useful in cases of blunt trauma, penetrating abdominal trauma, and chest deformities.

255. **The answer is E (all).** (Miller, 4/e. pp 1238, 2542.) High sympathetic blockade can block the cardiac accelerator fibers at T1–T4 and lead to bradycardia. All narcotics, except meperidine, cause bradycardia, probably through μ receptor stimulation. Vagal stimulation, such as pressure on the diaphragm, the carotid sinus, or the peritoneum, can also cause bradycardia. Pressure on the eyes can stimulate the oculocardiac reflex.

256. **The answer is C (2, 4).** (American Heart Association 1994 Text. pp. 1.29–1.32.) Bradycardia is defined as a heart rate less than 60 beats per minute. However, unless there are signs of poor cardiac output or poor peripheral perfusion—such as hypotension, unconsciousness, chest pain, or ectopic ventricular beats—there is no need to treat it. Initial treatment is with atropine 0.5 mg up to a total of 0.03 mg/kg. This can be followed, if necessary, by a transcutaneous pacemaker or dopamine or epinephrine infusions.

257. **The answer is C (2, 4).** Miller, 4/e. pp 2542–2553.) External or transvenous pacing should be instituted as soon as possible, although atropine and isoproterenol should be started in the meantime. Calcium is no longer recommended, because it has been shown to be of no proven benefit. However, it should be given whenever hyperkalemia is the etiology of the arrest. Atrial fibrillation and flutter often can be terminated by cardioversion at low energy levels, but if this is unsuccessful and the patient is doing poorly, incrementally higher energy levels should be attempted until the maximal level is reached. Atropine, lidocaine, and epinephrine can be given safely and effectively via the endotracheal tube.

258. **The answer is E (all).** (Miller, 4/e. p 1239.) Sinus tachycardias are usually due to sympathetic stimulation. This can be due to an inadequate level of anesthesia, hypovolemia, hypoxia, hypercarbia, hyperthermia, and sympathomimetic drugs. Less common causes include heart failure. The recommended treatment is to find and treat the underlying cause of the problem rather than the dysrhythmia itself.

259. **The answer is C (2, 4).** (Miller, 4/e. pp 1241–1242.) These supraventricular rhythms usually occur with preexisting cardiac disease. They are seen in patients with mitral valve disease, coronary artery disease, pulmonary embolism, cardiac trauma, and hyperthyroidism. Initially, the physiologic impairment consists of inadequate ventricular filling resulting from the rapid heart rate, which may compromise cardiac output. In patients with atrial fibrillation, the loss of atrial systole also may compromise LV filling.

260. **The answer is C (2, 4).** (Miller, 4/e. p 1242.) PVCs can be caused by many conditions. Electrolyte disturbances, hypoxemia, hypercarbia, bradycardia, and drug interactions as well as ischemia can all lead to PVCs. Premature atrial contractions with aberrant conduction can mimic PVCs and often are difficult to differentiate. PVCs should be investigated as to their cause, and the underlying cause should be treated. Multifocal beats, more than six per minute, and R-on-T phenomena are the types that most often lead to ventricular tachycardia and fibrillation.

261. **The answer is C (2, 4).** (Miller, 3/e. pp 2545–2547.) Atropine is not recommended as a treatment for stable ventricular tachycardia. The advanced cardiac life support (ACLS) protocol recommends lidocaine as the initial drug of choice. Procainamide or bretylium also may be used. Electrical cardioversion should be done if treatment with drugs fails in a stable patient or if the patient becomes unstable, such as the patient described in choice 3. The starting dose is 100 joule. After successful treatment, an infusion of whichever drug worked to suppress the rhythm should be started.

262. **The answer is B (1, 3).** (Miller, 4/e. pp 2552–2553.) PEA is a terminal rhythm that has a number of reversible causes. They include severe hypoxemia, acidosis, hypovolemia, pneumothorax, pericardial tamponade, and pulmonary embolism. There is no reason for electrical cardioversion, since electrical function is intact. Epinephrine is the most useful agent.

263. **The answer is C (2, 4).** (Stoelting, *Anesthesia and Co-Existing Disease,* 3/e. p 62.) Phenytoin's use as a dysrhythmic drug is limited to treating digitalis-induced dysrhythmias and in torsade des pointes, which has a prolonged Q-T interval. It does not cause the release of catecholamines.

264. **The answer is D (4).** (American Heart Association, 1994 Guidelines. p 3-3.) There is no effective cardiac output with ventricular fibrillation and therefore no pulse. The pattern on ECG is irregular and bizarre, with coarse, large depolarizations being seen first. These are easier to convert than is the fine ventricular fibrillation that eventually occurs.

265. The answer is E (all). (Barash, 3/e. p 1011.) The Valsalva maneuver involves the voluntary closure of the glottis and a forced expiration to increase intrathoracic pressure. During a Valsalva maneuver, venous pressures of the head and upper extremities increase, with a decrease in venous return to the right side of the heart. Cardiac output and blood pressure both decrease, resulting in a reflex increase in heart rate. After a Valsalva maneuver, there is a sudden increase in venous return to the right side of the heart with a subsequent increase in cardiac output and blood pressure; this then elicits a reflex bradycardia.

266. The answer is E (all). (Barash, 3/e. pp 816–817.) Coronary circulation receives approximately 5 percent of the cardiac output. Coronary flow decreases from epicardium to endocardium. The perfusion of myocardium occurs mostly during diastole. Flow through the left coronary artery occurs primarily during diastole, while flow through the right artery occurs during systole and diastole. Within the coronary perfusion pressure range of 50 to 120 mmHg, there is autoregulation of coronary flow. The most important regulators of coronary vascular tone are metabolic factors.

267. The answer is A (1, 2, 3). (Stoelting, *Pharmacology,* 2/e. pp 662–664.) Blood pressure is proportional to resistance to blood flow. Resistance to blood flow is greatest in the arterioles, where a large blood pressure drop—from approximately 85 to 30 mmHg—occurs. At the incisura in the tracing, left ventricular pressure declines and blood momentarily flows backward in the aorta and closes the aortic valve. The converting factor is 1 mmHg = 1.36 cmH$_2$O, and so 10 cm × 1 mmHg/1.36 cmH$_2$O = 7 mmHg. Pulse pressure is the difference between systolic and diastolic blood pressure. Pulse pressure is augmented as it travels through the arterial tree. This is due to decreasing arterial compliance in distal compared with central arteries as well as augmentation of pressure waves as a result of reflected waves from the periphery.

268. The answer is C (2, 4). (Miller, 4/e. pp 644–645.) Because the left-sided myocardium is maximally squeezed during systole, coronary perfusion occurs here primarily in diastole, but the right side is perfused during both systole and diastole. Coronary flow reserve is defined as the difference between resting and maximal coronary blood flow. Anything that causes a decrease in maximal blood flow, such as tachycardia, increased contractility, and increased ventricular size, will decrease coronary flow reserves. Autoregulation, or the maintenance of a constant blood flow over a range of perfusion pressures, does occur in the heart, but the range is from 50 to 120 mmHg. Many factors are thought to affect coronary vascular tone, but adenosine seems to be the most important. It is a local mediator which couples blood flow to oxygen consumption.

269. The answer is A (1, 2, 3). (Barash, 3/e. p 297.) Nifedipine is not available for intravenous administration. However, it is a potent vasodilator used in the treatment of

Prinzmetal angina (coronary vasospasm) and hypertension. Sublingually, it can immediately reverse these problems. Reflex tachycardia may result from vasodilation, and an increased cardiac output may result from the decrease in afterload.

270. **The answer is C (2, 4).** (Barash, 3/e. pp 1269–1270.) Cyclosporine inhibits activation of T-helper cells and decreases lymphokine production. It has hepato- and nephrotoxicity but is not toxic to marrow. Its nephrotoxicity is related to its effect on reducing renal blood flow (glomerular filtration rate). Mild hypertension can occur due to chronic toxic effects to the kidneys. There is usually an increase in BUN and creatinine as well as increased vulnerability to acute insults. Cyclosporine also promotes gingival hyperplasia.

271. **The answer is A (1, 2, 3).** (Miller, 4/e. pp 1791–1792.) Clotting during bypass is a lethal complication for the patient. The initial dose of heparin should be 300 to 400 units per kilogram body weight, and the ACT should be maintained above 400 s for the duration of the bypass. Any sign of clot should be treated immediately with more heparin. Inadequate heparinization also can lead to the consumption of clotting factors, leading to coagulopathic bleeding.

272. **The answer is E (all).** (Miller, 4/e. p 1792.) Many physiologic changes that are associated with bypass must be closely monitored. Problems such as malpositioning of the aortic cannula, aortic dissection, and oxygenator failure can cause acute decompensation in the patient.

273. **The answer is B (1, 3).** (Miller, 4/e. pp 1815–1818.) Blalock-Taussig shunts are systemic pulmonary arterial shunts created to improve pulmonary blood flow in patients with cyanotic heart disease secondary to decreased pulmonary blood flow. Tetralogy of Fallot and pulmonary atresia are cyanotic lesions that may require Blalock-Taussig shunts. Atrioventricular canal and Ebstein's anomaly are not cyanotic lesions.

274. **The answer is A (1, 2, 3).** (Miller, 4/e. p 1792.) Venous blood traverses the tubing via a siphon effect; air in the tubing creates obstruction to flow. Gravity dictates venous return, and so the greater the difference in height between the vena cava and the venous return reservoir, the greater the blood return.

275. **The answer is E (all).** (Stoelting, *Anesthesia and Co-Existing Disease*, 3/e. pp 28–34.) In mitral regurgitation, regurgitant flow also correlates with the intensity of the murmur. Forward flow is maximized and regurgitant flow is minimized with low systemic vascular resistance. Mild tachycardia reduces diastolic filling time and minimizes regurgitant flow. Right-sided cardiac output will accurately reflect left-sided output in mitral regurgitation as long as the aortic valve is competent.

276.   The answer is C (2, 4). (Stoelting, *Anesthesia and Co-Existing Disease*, 3/e. pp 24–28.) Elevations of pulmonary vascular resistance can precipitate right-sided heart failure. These patients already have elevated pulmonary vascular resistance and often pulmonary hypertension. Avoidance of high airway pressures, acidosis, and hypoxemia to minimize pulmonary vascular resistance is imperative. Heart rate should be kept normal. Tachycardia is especially detrimental because it impedes diastolic filling of an already underloaded left ventricle and reduces cardiac output. LV dysfunction is rare in pure lesions, as the ventricle is generally underloaded. Left atrial pressures increase as the disease progresses.

277.   The answer is C (2, 4). (Stoelting, *Anesthesia and Co-Existing Disease*, 3/e. pp 34–35.) Pulmonary hypertension and any disease process which overloads the right ventricle can lead to ventricular dilation and tricuspid regurgitation. Infectious causes of valvular failure are often associated with IV drug abuse. Anesthetic management includes maintaining right heart volume in the high normal range to keep stroke volume up. Nitrous oxide, hypercarbia, and hypoxemia can worsen pulmonary hypertension, increasing regurgitation. Inhalational agents tend to dilate the pulmonary vasculature, unloading the right heart.

278.   The answer is A (1, 2, 3). (Stoelting, *Anesthesia and Co-Existing Disease*, 3/e. pp 508–509.) Anaphylactic and anaphylactoid reactions have been associated with protamine administration, most often in patients taking insulin preparations that contain protamine and in patients allergic to seafood, as protamine is derived from salmon sperm. Histamine release, especially if the infusion is rapid, and pulmonary hypertension also have been associated with protamine infusion. Ventricular arrhythmias have not been linked specifically to protamine.

279.   The answer is E (all). (Stoelting, *Pharmacology*, 2/e. pp 468–469.) Heparin acutely displaces alkaline drugs from their binding sites. Drugs such as propranolol and diazepam may have higher serum levels in the presence of heparin. Heparin comes from animal tissue, making it a potential allergen. Rapid infusion of high doses of heparin may reduce MAP as a result of the relaxing effect of heparin on vascular smooth muscle. Thrombocytopenia can be seen in patients after about a week of therapy with heparin. This is thought to be due to either platelet aggregation or antiplatelet antibodies triggered by the heparin.

280.   The answer is D (4). (Stoelting, *Pharmacology*, 2/e. pp 469–470.) Heparin resistance secondary to low antithrombin III levels may be overcome by transfusing FFP, which restores antithrombin III levels to normal.

281.   The answer is E (all). (Barash, 3/e. pp 820–822.) With the opening of the mitral valve at point A, the ventricle begins to fill. Point B represents mitral valve closure and end-diastolic volume. At this time, contraction of the left ventricle with a closed mitral and aortic valve results in increased LV pressure without changes in volume (i.e, there is volumetric contraction). When LV pressure exceeds the aortic pressure at point C, the aortic valve opens and ventricular ejection begins. At point D the aortic valve closes, systole ceases, and the remaining volume is termed *end-systolic volume.* The decrease in LV pressure between points D and A without a change in LV volume is termed *isovolumetric relaxation.*

282. **The answer is C (2, 4).** (Stoelting, *Anesthesia and Co-Existing Disease,* 3/e. pp 63–66.) The "ground plate" should be placed as far as possible from the pulse generator. A low electrocautery current is less likely to be sensed by the pulse generator. Short bursts of the electrocautery 10 s apart minimize the chance of pacemaker malfunction. Myopotentials generated as a result of fasciculation may be interpreted as R waves and thus potentially inhibit the generator. Therefore, a defasciculating dose of muscle relaxant is necessary.

283. **The answer is E (all).** (Stoelting, *Anesthesia and Co-Existing Disease,* 3/e. pp 63–66.) The reason for placement, the date of placement, and the type of generator are all necessary preoperative information in a patient with an artificial cardiac pacemaker. The fixed rate of a VOO (asynchronous) pacemaker is 70 to 72 beats per minute; this is also the rate of a VVI pacemaker that is uninhibited. A chest x-ray may be useful in detecting a break in the pacemaker electrode.

284. **The answer is E (all).** (Stoelting, *Anesthesia and Co-existing Disease,* 3/e. pp. 63–66.) With judicious placement and low-density current, there is minimal skeletal muscle and cutaneous stimulation. NTPs are generally tolerated by awake patients with minimal sedation.

285. **The answer is D (4).** (Stoelting, *Anesthesia and Co-Existing Disease,* 3/e. pp 63–66.) Terms applied to a VOO pacemaker include *fixed rate* and *asynchronous.* VVI pacemakers are referred to as *demand, synchronous,* or *noncompetitive.* The first letter refers to the chamber paced, the second to the chamber sensed, and the third to the response of the generator to a sensed R or P wave. Hence, DVI implies that both atrium and ventricle are paced, the ventricle only is sensed, and the generator responds in an inhibitory fashion. (Remember, *P* [paced] comes before *S* [sensed] in the alphabet, as it does in pacemaker nomenclature.) A DDD pacemaker is designed to have the atrium and ventricle contract in sequence. The so-called atrial kick can add 20 to 30 percent to cardiac output, which may be crucial in some patients.

RESPIRATORY SYSTEM

Directions: Each question below contains five suggested responses. Select the **one best** response to each question.

286. A true statement about the Univent bronchial blocker tube is

(A) it is more difficult to place than a conventional double-lumen tube

(B) it is recommended that the tube be changed to a single-lumen tube for postoperative ventilation

(C) the tube allows for rapid deflation of the selected lung

(D) the bronchial blocker lumen is rarely blocked by secretions

(E) single lobes may be collapsed instead of an entire lung

287. A patient presents for excision of a bronchopleural cutaneous fistula. Which mode of intubation will most effectively achieve lung separation?

(A) Single-lumen endotracheal tube

(B) Single-lumen endotracheal tube and bronchial blocker

(C) Endobronchial intubation with a single-lumen tube

(D) Spontaneous mask ventilation

(E) Double-lumen endotracheal tube

288. A true statement about ventilation and perfusion of the lung is

- (A) ventilation and perfusion are most closely matched in West's zone 1
- (B) intrapleural pressure is more negative at the bottom of the upright lung than at the top
- (C) physiologic shunting is most pronounced in zone 2 of the lung
- (D) blood flow through zone 2 of the lung is dependent on the pressure difference between the arteries and the alveoli
- (E) zone 3 has the highest V/Q ratio of all the lung zones

289. Matching of ventilation and perfusion in the lung occurs best when the patient is in the

- (A) lateral decubitus position (LDP), awake, with closed chest
- (B) LDP, anesthetized, with closed chest
- (C) LDP, anesthetized, with open chest
- (D) LDP, anesthetized, paralyzed, with open chest
- (E) supine position, anesthetized, with closed chest

Directions: Each question below contains four suggested responses of which **one or more** is correct. Select:

(A)	if	**1, 2, and 3**	are correct
(B)	if	**1 and 3**	are correct
(C)	if	**2 and 4**	are correct
(D)	if	**4**	is correct
(E)	if	**1, 2, 3, and 4**	are correct

290. True statements regarding physiologic dead space include that it

(1) is the sum of alveolar and anatomic dead spaces
(2) can be assessed by the difference between end-tidal and arterial CO_2
(3) may be increased with large tidal volume positive pressure ventilation
(4) usually constitutes approximately 20 to 40 percent of tidal ventilation

291. In the preoperative evaluation of a patient for pneumonectomy, predictors of good postoperative function include

(1) FEV_1 greater than 2 L with an FEV/FVC ratio of 50 percent
(2) maximum oxygen uptake during exercise of 20 mL/kg or more
(3) selective pulmonary artery occlusion pressure of <35 mmHg
(4) postoperative FEV_1 of at least 600 mL

292. Anatomic shunts may be characterized by which of the following statements?

(1) They are approximately 10 percent of total cardiac output in normal persons
(2) They are increased in patients with cyanotic congenital heart disease
(3) They are normal or decreased in cirrhotic patients
(4) They are the result of direct emptying of pleural, bronchial, and thebesian veins into the left atrium

293. To calculate the physiologic shunt, it is useful to know which of the following?

(1) Mixed venous O_2
(2) Pa_{O_2}
(3) Hemoglobin
(4) Pa_{CO_2}

294. Hypoxic pulmonary vasoconstriction (HPV) is a normal autoregulatory mechanism to reduce blood flow to hypoventilated lung areas. True statements about HPV include

(1) it can be increased by low total FI_{O_2}
(2) prostaglandins increase HPV
(3) low Va/Q promotes HPV
(4) pulmonary vasodilators increase Pa_{O_2} in the presence of HPV

295. True statements about double-lumen tubes (DLTs) include which of the following?

   (1)   They may be useful in the repair of bronchopleural fistulae to isolate the lung
   (2)   The smallest DLT that will maintain good ventilation is the best tube to use
   (3)   Though both right- and left-sided DLTs can be used to collapse the left lung, left-sided tubes are used almost exclusively
   (4)   Fiberoptic bronchoscopy reveals that less than 30 percent of DLTs are malpositioned by clinical signs alone

296. True statements with regard to concentration effect include

   (1)   concentration effect means the inspired concentration of a given gas may influence both the alveolar concentration reached and the rate at which that concentration is reached
   (2)   concentration effect on a second gas when it is given concomitantly is termed the *second gas effect*
   (3)   two factors in the concentration effect are the effect of concentrating and the effect of augmenting the inspired ventilation
   (4)   concentration effect can be thought of as effectively increasing solubility with an increased concentration of inspired gas

297. True statements concerning going from two-lung to one-lung ventilation include

   (1)   in patients with normal preoperative pulmonary function (i.e., normal exercise capacity, normal pulmonary function tests), the alveolar-arterial difference for oxygen tension (A-a D_{O_2}) does not change
   (2)   if deterioration in Pa_{O_2} occurs, the use of vasoconstrictor drugs is likely to help restore Pa_{O_2} by increasing cardiac output and thereby blood flow to all parts of the lungs
   (3)   the change in arterial CO_2 is greater than that in arterial Pa_{O_2}
   (4)   pulmonary vascular resistance increases in the nondependent lung, which helps maintain Pa_{O_2}

298. True statements about pulmonary physiology include

   (1)   ventilation to the basilar regions of the normal lung is greater than that to the apical regions because of the greater compliance of the basilar alveoli
   (2)   a low cardiac output would be expected to increase West's zone 1 of the lung
   (3)   blood flow is greatest to basilar lung regions in a normal upright lung; however, the ratio of ventilation to perfusion is lower here than in apical regions
   (4)   the bases of normal upright lungs are better oxygenated than are the apices

SUMMARY OF DIRECTIONS

A	B	C	D	E
1,2,3	1,3	2,4	4	All are
only	only	only	only	correct

299. The following diagram depicts lung capacities and volumes. True statements about this diagram include

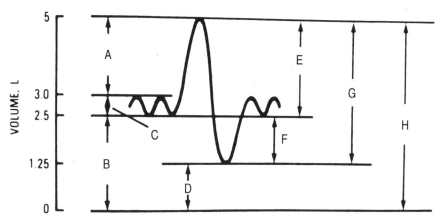

Adapted from Miller, *Anesthesia,* 4/e, with permission.

(1) arrow G describes vital capacity

(2) arrow B describes a lung volume that is reduced in all patients undergoing general anesthesia, whether breathing is controlled or spontaneous

(3) when closing capacity is less than the lung volume indicated by C, atelectasis will not occur

(4) the lung volume described by arrow G is reduced in patients with asthma

---

300. True statements concerning continuous positive airway pressure (CPAP) and positive end-expiratory pressure (PEEP) include

(1) CPAP can be delivered by nasal cannulae to newborns, but this is ineffective in adults

(2) CPAP and PEEP both increase functional residual capacity

(3) CPAP and PEEP can both worsen Pa_{O_2} in some situations

(4) an important benefit of CPAP and PEEP is that both can decrease the work of breathing

301. True statements about positive end-expiratory pressure (PEEP) include

(1) interstitial lung water is redistributed

(2) dead space ventilation may be increased

(3) functional residual capacity is increased

(4) pulmonary shunting may be increased

302. Physiologic changes associated with positive pressure ventilation include

    (1) reductions in cardiac output

    (2) increases in intracranial pressure (ICP)

    (3) decreases in portal vein blood flow

    (4) increases in urine volume and glomerular filtration rate (GFR)

303. Which of the following would be a normal value in a young, healthy subject?

    (1) Vital capacity of 60 to 70 mL/kg

    (2) Maximal expiratory pressure of 200 cmH_2O

    (3) Tidal volume of 7 mL/kg

    (4) Maximal inspiratory pressure of -25 cmH_2O

304. Which of the following will increase zone 1?

    (1) Oligemic shock

    (2) Pulmonary embolism

    (3) Positive pressure ventilation

    (4) Pulmonary hypertension

305. Hypoxic pulmonary vasoconstriction (HPV)

    (1) causes the greatest increase in Pa_{O_2} when the amount of hypoxic lung is less than 30 percent

    (2) is inhibited in vitro by halogenated anesthetics

    (3) is inhibited in animal models by thiopental

    (4) is not significantly affected by halogenated agents in humans undergoing one-lung ventilation

306. Pulmonary vascular resistance (PVR) is increased

    (1) by decreased cardiac output

    (2) by alveolar hypoxia

    (3) by hypercapnia

    (4) at functional residual capacity (FRC)

307. With regard to double-lumen endotracheal tubes,

    (1) a left-sided tube is more difficult to place properly than a right-sided tube

    (2) an absolute indication for placement is operative management of a bronchopleural fistula

    (3) they are too large to be used through a tracheostomy

    (4) they are relatively contraindicated in a patient with a full stomach

308. Ways to increase Pa_{O_2} during one-lung ventilation include

    (1) positive end-expiratory pressure (PEEP) to the dependent lung

    (2) continuous positive airway pressure (CPAP) to the nondependent lung

    (3) clamping of the pulmonary artery to the nondependent lung

    (4) adjustment of tidal ventilation to the dependent lung

309. Complications of mediastinoscopy include

    (1) hemorrhage

    (2) injury to the phrenic nerve

    (3) pneumothorax

    (4) hemiparesis

310. The head-down position during laparoscopy results in which of the following pulmonary changes?

   (1)   Decreased functional residual capacity and total lung volume

   (2)   Decreased pulmonary compliance

   (3)   Development of atelectasis

   (4)   More effective relationship of ventilation to perfusion

311. Risks of hyperoxia include

   (1)   retinopathy of prematurity (retrolental fibroplasia)

   (2)   ventilatory depression

   (3)   absorption atelectasis

   (4)   increased size of pneumothorax

SUMMARY OF DIRECTIONS

A	B	C	D	E
1,2,3	1,3	2,4	4	All are
only	only	only	only	correct

312. With regard to the work of breathing,

    (1)   oxygen utilization by the respiratory muscles in normal people at rest is 5 percent of total body oxygen utilization

    (2)   in patients with cardiopulmonary disease, resting oxygen utilization by the respiratory muscles is 25 percent of total body utilization

    (3)   in severe cardiopulmonary disease, the work of breathing is so high that it results in a net loss of oxygen

    (4)   the increased oxygen consumption in cardiorespiratory disease is due to the recruitment of other muscles

RESPIRATORY SYSTEM

ANSWERS

286. **The answer is E.** (Miller, 4/e. pp 1701–1702.) The Univent bronchial blocker has certain advantages over the conventional double-lumen tube. These include ease of placement, ventilation during placement of the blocker portion, easy use for postoperative ventilation, and selective collapse of lung segments, which may aid in maintenance of Pa_{O_2}. Disadvantages include the fact that the bronchial lumen is very small, causing deflation and inflation of the selected lung to be slow, and easy blockage by secretions.

287. **The answer is E.** (Miller, 4/e. p 1689.) Resection of a bronchopleural cutaneous fistula is an absolute indication for lung separation and placement of a double-lumen endotracheal tube because all ventilation may exit via the fistula. There are other methods of lung separation, but they are not as effective or safe as use of a double-lumen endotracheal tube. A single-lumen endotracheal tube or spontaneous mask ventilation will not achieve lung separation. An endobronchial intubation can be attempted, but there may be blockage of the right upper lobe, and continuous positive airway pressure (CPAP) cannot be applied to the nondependent lung. A single-lumen endotracheal tube and a bronchial blocker can be used. Pitfalls with this technique include difficulty placing the blocker and movement and malposition of the blocker and tube.

288. **The answer is D.** (Barash, 3/e. pp 757–758.) In the upright lung, ventilation and perfusion are most closely matched in zone 2, the midsection of the lung. Here blood flow is dependent on Ppa-PA, not on venous pressure. Intrapleural pressure is more negative at the apices of the lung compared with the bottom. Zone 3, the base of the upright lung, has the least amount of physiologic shunt and the lowest V/Q ratio because of high perfusion. Perfusion is dictated primarily by gravity.

128   **ANESTHESIOLOGY**

289. **The answer is A.** (Miller, 4/e. pp 1685–1689.) In each scenario listed, perfusion remains gravity-dependent and is best in dependent areas of lung. Ventilation, however, matches perfusion only in an awake patient with closed chest in LDP. While abdominal contents result in a greater cephalad displacement of dependent diaphragm, this results in greater doming of the diaphragm and more efficient contraction of a spontaneously breathing patient. Induction of anesthesia results in loss of functional residual capacity (FRC) in both lungs. Loss in lung volume causes alveoli in each lung to occupy new positions on the compliance curve, with the result that the alveoli of the upper, nondependent lung are more compliant and receive more ventilation. In addition, the effect of compression by the hilum and abdominal contents further decreases lung volume. With the opening of the chest wall, total lung compliance is now the compliance of just the lung parenchyma, resulting in overinflation of the nondependent lung. Ventilation in the dependent lung is decreased. With paralysis, the dependent diaphragm moves further cephalad compared with the nondependent diaphragm.

290. **The answer is E (all).** (Barash, 3/e. pp 758–759.) By definition, dead space is air that does not participate in gas exchange.

291. **The answer is A (1, 2, 3).** (Miller, 4/e. p 899.) There are several phases to preoperative testing for a pneumonectomy candidate. Initial PFTs should show an FEV_1 of at least 2 L, MVV greater than 50 percent, and RV/TLC < 50 percent. Further tests are needed if these criteria are not met, including assessing individual lung ventilation and perfusion by spirometry and selective pulmonary artery occlusion. Postoperative lung FEV_1 must be at least 800 mL for successful ventilation. Exercise stress testing of lung function and oxygen consumption has become a useful tool as well.

292. **The answer is C (2, 4).** (Barash, 3/e. p 760.) Anatomic shunts are approximately 2 to 5 percent of total cardiac output in normal persons. They result from direct emptying of pleural, bronchial, and thebesian veins into the left atrium. Anatomic shunts are increased in patients with cyanotic congenital heart disease and those with advanced cirrhosis as a result of intrapulmonary arteriovenous anastomoses.

293. **The answer is E (all).** (Barash, 3/e. p 760.) Physiologic shunt, the ratio of shunted cardiac output to total cardiac output, may be defined as the ratio of the difference between pulmonary capillary oxygen content and arterial oxygen content over the difference between pulmonary capillary oxygen content and mixed venous oxygen content. The hemoglobin, oxygen saturation, and Pa_{O_2} are needed to calculate the arterial or mixed venous oxygen content. Pulmonary capillary oxygen content is derived from pulmonary capillary oxygen tension (Pa_{O_2}). The latter value is obtained from the ideal gas equation, which has Pa_{CO_2} as one of its variables.

294. **The answer is B (1, 3).** (Miller, 4/e. pp 583–584.) HPV works by increasing pulmonary vascular resistance in hypoxic areas of the lung. Prostaglandins tend to attenuate HPV, as they are pulmonary artery dilators. Pulmonary vasodilators decrease Pa_{O_2} in the face of significant HPV by reversing the process and sending blood flow back to hypoxemic areas.

295. **The answer is B (1, 3).** (Miller, 4/e. pp 1689–1696.) The largest DLT which can fit through the glottic opening is the best to use, as it facilitates ventilation and suctioning. Sizes range from 26 to 41 French. The right upper lobe is easy to compromise while one is using a right-sided DLT, and so left tubes are used almost exclusively today. Bronchoscopy reveals that nearly 78 percent of DLTs are malpositioned by clinical signs alone. Surgical positioning and manipulation can move the tubes around. If Pa_{O_2} is falling during one-lung ventilation, checking of tube position by fiberoptic bronchoscopy can be done easily.

296. **The answer is A (1, 2, 3).** (Miller, 4/e. p 105.) The concentration effect means that the inspired concentration of a given gas influences both the concentration at the alveoli and the rate of the attainment of the alveolar concentration. The concentrating effect and augmentation of inspired ventilation are two factors in the concentration effect. It can be thought of as a decrease in solubility with an increase in inspired concentration. "Overpressure" is a clinical application of the concentration effect. Concentration effect on a second gas when it is given concomitantly is termed the *second gas effect.*

297. **The answer is D (4).** (Miller, 4/e. pp 1705–1709.) Assumption of one-lung ventilation creates a large obligatory right-to-left shunt, which increases the A-a D_{O_2}. Vasoconstrictor drugs do not always improve cardiac output, but more important, they tend to vasoconstrict normoxic more than hypoxic lung areas, which diverts blood flow to the unventilated lung. Dopamine may have less of this effect than do other vasoconstrictors, making it a reasonable inotropic choice in patients with lung disease. This may further impair oxygenation. CO_2 is not appreciably affected by one-lung ventilation, since one lung can compensate for the unventilated lung by giving off more than the usual amount of CO_2. The same does not hold true for taking up oxygen in one ventilated lung versus two. The pulmonary vasculature responds to atelectasis and hypoxia with vasoconstriction (i.e., hypoxic pulmonary vasoconstriction). This diverts blood flow from the nondependent to the dependent lung, which helps minimize shunt.

298. **The answer is A (1, 2, 3).** (Miller, 4/e. pp 577–582.) Basilar alveoli are more compressed than are apical alveoli because of higher pleural pressure in lung bases. These small alveoli are more compliant than are larger apical alveoli and therefore receive a larger portion of tidal volume. In West's zone 1, alveolar pressure exceeds pulmonary arterial and venous pressures, and no blood flow takes place (dead space). Factors that increase alveolar pressure (such as positive pressure ventilation) or decrease arterial pressure (such as shock) increase zone 1. Both ventilation and perfusion increase as one moves from apical to basilar regions, but perfusion increases more than ventilation. Therefore, the V/Q ratio is highest at the apex. The higher V/Q of lung apices means better oxygenation in this area. For the same reason, lung bases are hypercarbic compared with apices.

299. **The answer is A (1, 2, 3).** (Miller, 4/e. p 590.) The change in lung volume from maximal expiration to maximal inspiration defines the vital capacity. Reduction of functional residual capacity occurs within 1 min of induction of general anesthesia, and the mechanism, although not clearly understood, is attributed to atelectasis, cephalad displacement of the diaphragm, reduction in outward recoil of the chest wall, and other factors. As long as closing capacity (the lung volume at which airways begin to close) remains below tidal volume (C), airways will remain open during normal breathing. The vital capacity, when measured as a forced maneuver (FVC), is normal in asthmatic patients, but the volume exhaled in the first second (FEV_1) is reduced in these patients.

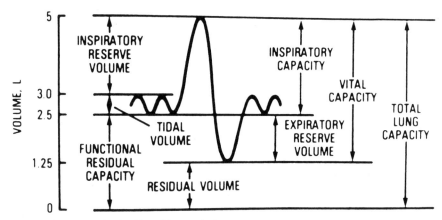

From Miller, *Anesthesia,* 4/e, with permission.

300. **The answer is E (all).** (Miller, 4/e. pp 2457–2458.) Nasal cannulae are effective in newborns because newborns breathe through the nose. Both CPAP and PEEP keep alveoli open at the end of expiration, which increases functional residual capacity. This converts atelectatic lung regions with severe ventilation-perfusion (V/Q) mismatching into areas of better V/Q match. These therapies can increase pulmonary vascular resistance and potentially shift blood away from well-ventilated areas, which promotes V/Q mismatch. Additionally, venous return to the heart can be impeded and thus reduce cardiac output, which also can lead to deterioration in Pa_{O_2}. By increasing lung volumes, these therapies improve lung compliance, which reduces the work of breathing.

301. **The answer is A (1, 2, 3).** (Miller, 4/e. pp 2418–2422.) PEEP increases oxygenation by two mechanisms. First, by shifting water from between the alveoli and capillaries to the peribronchial and hilar areas, gas exchange is facilitated. Second, by recruiting collapsed alveoli and increasing alveolar volumes, oxygenation may be improved. Excessive PEEP can cause a collapse of small vessels and lead to increased dead space, which will compromise oxygenation. PEEP decreases intrapulmonary shunting by recruiting collapsed alveoli.

302. **The answer is A (1, 2, 3).** (Miller, 4/e. pp 2425–2426.) Increased intrathoracic pressure from positive pressure ventilation will reduce venous return to the right side of the heart and lead to hypotension, but this can be prevented with volume loading. There is a risk of increasing ICP with positive pressure ventilation because rises in intrapleural pressure, which occur with positive pressure ventilation, may reduce cerebral outflow; this is a problem mainly in patients with poor cerebral compliance. Portal vein and renal blood flow are decreased. This may lead to hepatic dysfunction and decreases in urine volume and GFR.

303. **The answer is A (1, 2, 3).** (Miller, 4/e. p 886.) A vital capacity of 10 to 15 mL/kg is needed just for the work of breathing. Expiratory pressure is an indicator of the ability to cough. Normal inspiratory pressure is -125 cmH$_2$O, and this measurement correlates with the ability to take a deep breath.

304. **The answer is B (1, 3).** (Miller, 4/e. pp 578–579.) Zone 1 consists of an area where $P_A > P_{PA} > P_{PV}$ (P_A = alveolar pressure, P_{PA} = pulmonary artery pressure, P_{PV} = pulmonary venous pressure). The region functions as alveolar dead space, with no blood flow and therefore no gas exchange. Alveolar dead space or wasted ventilation increases with either a decrease in P_{PA} as is seen in oligemic shock or an increase in P_A as is seen during positive pressure ventilation. Pulmonary embolism and pulmonary hypertension both increase P_{PA}.

305. **The answer is C (2, 4).** (Miller, 4/e. pp 1678–1682.) The greatest increase in Pa$_{O_2}$ as a result of HPV occurs when 30 to 70 percent of the lung is made hypoxic. In vitro heart-lung preparations have demonstrated inhibition of HPV by halogenated anesthetics. No intravenous anesthetic has been shown to inhibit HPV. HPV is not significantly inhibited by halogenated anesthetics in humans undergoing one-lung ventilation.

306. **The answer is A (1, 2, 3).** (Miller, 4/e. pp 580–585.) Pressure equals flow times resistance. In the face of decreasing flow (cardiac output), pressure is maintained by increasing resistance. The increase of PVR by alveolar hypoxia is referred to as *hypoxic pulmonary vasoconstriction.* The net effect is to decrease blood flow to underventilated areas of the lung. PVR is lowest at FRC.

307. **The answer is C (2, 4).** (Miller, 4/e. p 1689.) A right-sided tube is more difficult to place correctly because of the variable location of the right upper lobe bronchus. Absolute indications may be divided into three categories: isolation of lungs to prevent cross contamination (e.g., hemorrhage), control of distribution of ventilation (e.g., bronchopleural fistula), and need for unilateral pulmonary lavage (e.g., pulmonary alveolar proteinosis). Double-lumen endotracheal tubes may be used through a tracheostomy, although the tracheal cuff may lie outside the trachea. With the risk of aspiration increasing with a full stomach, the somewhat technically more difficult double-lumen tube placement is relatively contraindicated.

308. **The answer is E (all).** (Miller, 4/e. pp 1709–1717.) PEEP to the dependent, ventilated lung can recruit alveoli and improve compliance. CPAP to the nonventilated, nondependent lung results in alveoli distended by oxygen that can participate in gas exchange. Clamping of the pulmonary artery to the nondependent lung decreases the amount of shunt substantially. Adjusting tidal volume to the dependent, ventilated lung is done to maximally decrease atelectasis in that lung while minimizing increases in pulmonary vascular resistance.

309. **The answer is E (all).** (Miller, 4/e. pp 1725–1728.) Mediastinoscopy, which usually is performed to help make the diagnosis of lung carcinoma, involves making an incision in the sternal notch and dissecting down to the mediastinum. Structures immediately adjacent to the mediastinoscope include the thoracic aorta, trachea, recurrent laryngeal nerve, superior vena cava, and innominate, left subclavian, and left common carotid arteries. Complications, in descending order of frequency, include hemorrhage, pneumothorax, recurrent laryngeal nerve injury, infection, wound tumor implantation, phrenic nerve injury, esophageal injury, chylothorax, air embolus, and hemiparesis.

310. **The answer is A (1, 2, 3).** (Miller, 4/e. p 2020.) The head-down position during laparoscopy combined with pneumoperitoneum induces a decrease in the ventilation to perfusion ratio which may predispose the patient to hypoxia. Lung volumes diminish for these two reasons, while pulmonary perfusion is maintained. Hypoxemia caused by this increased V/Q mismatch can be treated with positive end-expiratory pressure (PEEP).

311. **The answer is A (1, 2, 3).** (Miller, 4/e. pp 606–607, 614.) In premature infants whose gestational age is 44 weeks or less (the exact number of weeks is controversial), a Pa_{O_2} of >80 mmHg for 3 h or more can cause retinopathy of prematurity and blindness. Hyperoxia can suppress ventilation in patients who are dependent on the hypoxic drive to breathe. Absorption atelectasis occurs in areas of the lung with high V/Q ratios in patients who breathe enriched O_2 mixtures. Here the rapid rise in Pa_{O_2} can cause an influx of O_2 into the blood that exceeds the inflow of O_2 into alveoli, eventually causing alveolar shrinkage and collapse. Hyperoxia does not enlarge a pneumothorax.

312. **The answer is A (1, 2, 3).** (Miller, 4/e. pp 2405–2406.) The increased oxygen consumption in cardiorespiratory disease is due primarily to an increase in minute ventilation.

NEUROLOGY

Directions: Each question below contains five suggested responses. Select the **one best** response to each question.

313. Correct placement of a central venous catheter for treatment of a venous air embolus can be ascertained by all the following methods EXCEPT

(A) a radiograph of the chest

(B) configuration of the P waves on the electrocardiogram with a saline-filled catheter that acts as a unipolar lead

(C) inserting the central line to 5 cm and stopping

(D) discerning a transduced venous pressure waveform

(E) transducing the venous catheter while advancing it until right ventricular pressure patterns are seen and then pulling the catheter back until one sees a right atrial pressure pattern

314. Causes of pulmonary dysfunction after acute spinal cord transection in the cervical region include all the following EXCEPT

(A) impaired alveolar ventilation

(B) cervical cord transection in the C2–C4 region, which leads to diaphragmatic paralysis with apnea and death

(C) neurogenic pulmonary edema

(D) greatly diminished vital capacity

(E) restrictive lung changes that lead to an inability to clear bronchial secretions

315. Treatment of a venous air embolus includes all the following EXCEPT

 (A) irrigation of the operative site by the surgeon and application of bone wax to all bone edges to seal open vessels

 (B) discontinuation of nitrous oxide (N_2O) if it is being used and increasing the FI_{O_2} to 1.0

 (C) attempting to aspirate the venous air embolus from the right heart via a central line

 (D) administration of mannitol 0.25 g/kg both to decrease intracranial pressure and for renal protection

 (E) support of the cardiovascular system with fluid administration and an inotrope if necessary

316. True statements concerning EEG patterns and their relationships to various anesthetic agents include all the following EXCEPT

 (A) isoflurane at 2.0 to 2.5 MAC causes electrical silence

 (B) barbiturates produce electrical silence

 (C) enflurane at 2.0 MAC causes seizure activity

 (D) high-dose fentanyl causes seizure activity

 (E) halothane, even in high doses, rarely causes electrical silence

317. With normocapnia, all the following drugs increase the intracranial pressure (ICP) EXCEPT

 (A) ketamine

 (B) lidocaine

 (C) N_2O

 (D) halothane

 (E) isoflurane

318. All the following statements regarding intracranial pressure are true EXCEPT

 (A) normal intracranial pressure is 10 to 15 mmHg

 (B) intracranial pressure increases lead to decreased cerebral perfusion pressure

 (C) plateau waves are decreases in intracranial pressure seen after mannitol diuresis

 (D) pretreatment with a nondepolarizing muscle relaxant prevents the rise in intracranial pressure seen with succinylcholine

 (E) the supine position increases intracranial pressure

319. True statements concerning the use of succinylcholine in patients with spinal cord injuries include all the following EXCEPT

 (A) nonparalyzing doses of a nondepolarizing muscle relaxant will attenuate the risk of hyperkalemia after administration of succinylcholine

 (B) the cause of hyperkalemia in response to the use of succinylcholine may be a proliferation of extrajunctional acetylcholine receptors

 (C) peak release of potassium after succinylcholine occurs when the injury is about 14 days old

 (D) hyperkalemia seen after the use of succinylcholine is not dependent on the dose

 (E) if at all possible, the use of succinylcholine should be avoided

320. From fastest onset of action to slowest onset of action, the modalities for decreasing intracranial pressure are

(A) hyperventilation, osmotic diuretics, loop diuretics, steroids
(B) hyperventilation, osmotic diuretics, steroids, loop diuretics
(C) hyperventilation, loop diuretics, osmotic diuretics, steroids
(D) loop diuretics, hyperventilation, osmotic diuretics, steroids
(E) loop diuretics, osmotic diuretics, hyperventilation, steroids

321. Which of the following agents is most likely to modify autoregulation of cerebral blood flow in response to changes in arterial blood pressure?

(A) Thiopental
(B) Fentanyl
(C) Morphine
(D) Halothane
(E) Isoflurane

322. Correct statements concerning monitoring for a venous air embolus with the use of a precordial Doppler probe include

(A) correct positioning of the Doppler probe is usually to the left lower end of the sternum down to the xiphoid process
(B) correct positioning of the Doppler probe is usually to the left of the sternum between the third and sixth intercostal spaces
(C) confirmation of correct positioning of the Doppler probe occurs when the second heart sound is the loudest
(D) confirmation of correct positioning of the Doppler probe occurs when 5 to 10 mL of crystalloid solution is injected through a central line and a loud roaring sound is heard
(E) air emboli as small as 0.02 mL can be detected by a sound change

323. The most sensitive means of detection of a venous air embolism is

(A) end-tidal CO_2
(B) Doppler probe
(C) pulmonary arterial catheter
(D) transesophageal echo
(E) pulse oximetry

324. The complication most commonly associated with the sitting position is

(A) compression injury
(B) marked postural hypotension
(C) quadriplegia
(D) Doppler-detectable venous air embolism
(E) subdural hematoma

Directions: Each question below contains four suggested responses of which **one or more** is correct. Select

(A)	if	**1, 2, and 3**	are correct
(B)	if	**1 and 3**	are correct
(C)	if	**2 and 4**	are correct
(D)	if	**4**	is correct
(E)	if	**1, 2, 3, and 4**	are correct

325. True statements about the management of patients with elevated intracranial pressure include

(1) etomidate is contraindicated as an induction agent because it can produce seizures

(2) PEEP would be expected to have a beneficial influence on cerebral perfusion pressure

(3) succinylcholine is absolutely contraindicated because fasciculations are likely to increase intracranial pressure

(4) hyperventilation to a Pa_{CO_2} of 20 torr is associated with a reduction in cerebral blood flow of 50 percent

326. True statements about the sitting position include

(1) the patient's chin should be just touching the chest

(2) positive end-expiratory pressure can increase right atrial pressure and cause a paradoxical air embolus through a patent foramen ovale

(3) postoperative visual field defects and, in rare cases, blindness are the most serious complications of brainstem edema from posterior fossa surgery

(4) the potential for circulatory instability, due to poor venous return to the heart, is an important concern

327. Regarding venous air embolism in patients undergoing craniotomy in the sitting position,

(1) a Doppler probe should be positioned to the left of the sternum between the third and sixth intercostal spaces

(2) a mill-wheel murmur is quite specific for venous air embolism but is not sensitive

(3) the first thing that should be done when a venous air embolus is suspected is to place the patient in a supine position to prevent further entrainment of air

(4) nitrous oxide should be discontinued promptly to avoid increasing the size of the venous air bubbles

328. Dangerous sequelae of a venous air embolus (VAE) include

(1) acute cor pulmonale and resultant cardiovascular collapse

(2) refractory arterial hypoxemia resulting from obstruction of flow from the right ventricle

(3) paradoxical air embolus through a probe-patent foramen ovale to the cerebral and coronary vasculature

(4) acute onset of disseminated intravascular coagulation (DIC)

329. True statements regarding autonomic hyperreflexia include

(1) it is rare in a spinal cord injury below level T4

(2) regional anesthesia is protective against this response

(3) beta blockers given perioperatively protect against this response

(4) bradycardia is one of the hallmarks of the response

330. Appropriate concerns in anesthetizing a patient who sustained a spinal cord injury at T5 4 days ago include

(1) the possibility of bradycardia and cardiac arrest on tracheal suctioning

(2) avoidance of succinylcholine

(3) loss of temperature regulation

(4) the possibility of severe hypertension and bradycardia (i.e., autonomic hyperreflexia) during cystoscopic procedures

331. Signs of autonomic hyperreflexia include

(1) hypertension

(2) tachycardia

(3) vasodilation above the spinal cord lesion that leads to nasal stuffiness and flushing

(4) vasodilation below the spinal cord lesion that leads to urinary incontinence and flushing

332. True statements concerning anesthetic management in patients with spinal cord transection for genitourinary (GU) procedures include

(1) general anesthesia will adequately prevent autonomic hyperreflexia

(2) local anesthesia will adequately prevent autonomic hyperreflexia

(3) spinal anesthesia will adequately prevent autonomic hyperreflexia

(4) no anesthesia is necessary

333. True statements pertaining to EEG patterns include

(1) hypocarbia may cause seizure foci and increase EEG activity

(2) hypercarbia slows EEG activity

(3) hypoxia slows EEG activity

(4) severe hypotension is needed before significant changes are seen

334. Electroconvulsive therapy (ECT) is deemed successful if

(1) there is a grand mal seizure lasting 25 to 60 s

(2) the patient tolerates at least 60 V

(3) an EEG pattern demonstrates a grand mal seizure

(4) the patient has memory loss after ECT

335. Physiologic side effects of electroconvulsive therapy (ECT) include

(1) stimulation of the parasympathetic nervous system

(2) loss of bladder and bowel control

(3) stimulation of the sympathetic nervous system

(4) post-ECT ileus

336. ECT is contraindicated in patients

    (1)   with orthopedic prostheses
    (2)   after heart transplantation
    (3)   with transvenous pacemakers
    (4)   with increased intracranial pressure (ICP)

337. The indications for ECT include

    (1)   organic mental syndrome
    (2)   severe anxiety
    (3)   anorexia nervosa
    (4)   severe mental depression

338. In a patient with suspected intracranial hypertension, which of the following induction agents should be avoided?

    (1)   Morphine
    (2)   Isoflurane
    (3)   Valium
    (4)   Ketamine

339. Which of the following agents will cause an increase in CSF production?

    (1)   Halothane
    (2)   Isoflurane
    (3)   Ketamine
    (4)   Enflurane

NEUROLOGY

ANSWERS

313. **The answer is C.** (Stoelting, *Anesthesia and Co-Existing Disease,* 3/e. p 193.) Placing a central line for a sitting position procedure is advantageous not only for treatment of a venous air embolus with aspiration but also as a monitoring tool for fluid therapy. A venous air embolus can be treated by placing the catheter in the right atrium to remove the air. Placement can be monitored in several ways. A chest radiograph may be taken. The central line filled with saline as a unipolar ECG lead may be used until biphasic P waves are seen, although this method puts the patient at risk for microshock hazard. One may transduce a venous pressure wave or transduce the catheter while it is advanced until a right ventricular wave pattern is seen and then pull the catheter back until a right atrial wave pattern is seen. If the catheter is inserted only 5 cm from any insertion point, it will be well outside the central circulation and nowhere near the right atrium.

314. **The answer is C.** (Stoelting, *Anesthesia and Co-Existing Disease,* 3/e. p 226.) During the initial phase of acute cervical cord transection, the major cause of morbidity and mortality is pulmonary dysfunction. If the transection is through the C2–C4 level, the diaphragm is paralyzed by phrenic nerve dysfunction, leading to apnea and death. Even if the diaphragm is intact and the patient has a normal tidal volume (transection at C6–C7), there will still be restrictive changes with decreases in FEV, FVC, and FRC. The patient will be unable to clear secretions or protect the airway, and atelectasis and pneumonia may result. Neurogenic pulmonary edema is a not a problem.

315. **The answer is D.** (Stoelting, *Anesthesia and Co-Existing Disease,* 3/e. pp 195–196.) Irrigating the operative field and sealing the bone edges prevent further entrainment of air. N_2O may increase the size of the embolus, and so it should be discontinued. If a central line has been placed, it may be possible to aspirate the air through it from the right heart. The cardiovascular system should be supported, but mannitol is of no help in this situation.

316. **The answer is D.** (Miller, 4/e. pp 1322–1325.) High-dose fentanyl does not cause seizure activity to appear on the EEG. As the dose of fentanyl increases, there is a progression to a slower EEG pattern. With administration of 30 to 70 mg/kg, there is a theta pattern.

317. **The answer is B.** (Miller, 4/e. pp 1919–1921.) Ketamine increases cerebral blood flow and the cerebral metabolic rate. Along with etomidate and thiopental, lidocaine is a cerebral vasoconstrictor. Halothane and isoflurane will not increase ICP if the patient is hyperventilated.

318. **The answer is C.** (Miller, 4/e. pp 1909–1917.) Since cerebral perfusion pressure (CPP) is equal to arterial pressure (AP) minus intracranial pressure (ICP), increases in ICP decrease CPP. Plateau waves are abrupt increases in ICP that last 10 to 15 min. Increased cerebral blood flow is thought to be the cause. Increased cerebral venous pressure will increase ICP. Therefore, patients with increased ICP should be nursed in the head-up position.

319. **The answer is A.** (Stoelting, *Anesthesia and Co-Existing Disease,* 3/e. p 229.) Succinylcholine can cause precipitous increases in serum potassium levels in patients with spinal cord injuries. A possible mechanism may be the proliferation of extrajunctional acetylcholine receptor sites below the spinal cord lesion. Safe periods for the use of succinylcholine are vague, and administration of nondepolarizing muscle relaxants before succinylcholine will not reliably prevent hyperkalemia. Hyperkalemia is not a dose-dependent phenomenon. If at all possible, succinylcholine should be avoided in patients with spinal cord injuries.

320. **The answer is A.** (Miller, 4/e. pp 1913–1917.) Hyperventilation works immediately. Osmotic diuretics begin to lower ICP in about 15 min, whereas loop diuretics lower ICP in 30 to 45 min. Steroids take hours before they begin to lower ICP.

321. **The answer is D.** (Miller, 4/e. pp 697–709.) Halothane is the most potent cerebral vasodilator among all the inhalational anesthetics. Although CO_2 responsiveness apparently remains intact, autoregulation of cerebral blood flow in response to changes in arterial blood pressure is impaired with inhalational agents. In particular, it is more impaired with the anesthetics that have the greatest cerebral vasodilatory effect.

322. **The answer is D.** (Stoelting, *Anesthesia and Co-Existing Disease,* 3/e. p 194.) Precordial Doppler monitoring is useful for detection of venous air emboli during sitting craniotomies. The correct position of the probe is to the right of the sternum between the third and sixth interspaces. Confirmation is achieved by injection of 5 to 10 mL of a crystalloid solution into a central line, which will be heard as a loud roaring sound. An air embolus as small as 0.25 mL may be picked up with the Doppler probe as a sound change. The precordial Doppler probe and the transesophageal echo are the two most sensitive monitors for venous air emboli.

323. The answer is D. (Miller, 4/e. pp 1903–1904.) Methods of detection of a venous air embolism in declining order of sensitivity are transesophageal echo, Doppler probe, end-tidal CO_2, and pulmonary arterial catheter. Decreased oxygen saturation as noted by pulse oximetry is a late sign.

324. The answer is D. (Miller, 4/e. pp 1065–1070.) Compression injuries are rare, and quadriplegia is a very rare complication. More than one-third of patients experience transient and mild postural hypotension. Hemodynamically significant circulatory instability occurs in only 3 to 5 percent of patients in the sitting position. Doppler-detectable venous air embolism occurs with an incidence of 25 to 50 percent in patients in the sitting position.

325. The answer is D (4). (Miller, 4/e. pp 1909–1917.) Etomidate does not produce seizures; it can cause clonic movements, but those movements do not represent seizure activity. PEEP can worsen intracranial hypertension. Succinylcholine can increase intracranial pressure, but the cause is unclear. Pretreatment with a nondepolarizing muscle relaxant can attenuate this response.

326. The answer is C (2, 4). (Miller, 4/e. pp 1065–1070. Stoelting, *Pharmacology,* 3/e. p 194.) Hyperflexion of the neck can impede venous drainage from the head and result in tongue and facial swelling. Allow one to two fingerbreadths between the chin and chest to avoid this complication. A substantial proportion of the population has a patent foramen ovale. Positive end-expiratory pressure or a Valsalva maneuver can shunt right atrial air into the left heart and the systemic circulation. Brainstem edema is a dangerous complication of posterior fossa surgery but manifests as disturbances in swallowing and breathing and circulatory instability. Legs should be wrapped while the patient is supine to avoid the complication of circulatory instability.

327. The answer is C (2, 4). (Stoelting, *Pharmacology,* 3/e. p 195.) Doppler placement is to the right of the sternum between the third and sixth intercostal spaces. The murmur is quite specific for a venous air embolus but is not at all sensitive. Nitrous oxide, if used, should be stopped; the surgeon should be informed so that he or she can flood the operative field, the neck veins should be compressed, and air should be aspirated from the right atrial catheter, if one is being used. Valuable time should not be lost in first trying to change the patient's position.

328. The answer is A (1, 2, 3). (Stoelting, *Anesthesia and Co-Existing Disease,* 3/e. pp 194–195.) The exact reason why a VAE causes cardiovascular collapse is unknown. It is hypothesized that the VAE causes obstruction of right ventricular outflow, which leads to acute cor pulmonale and arterial hypoxemia. Dead space ventilation increases, pulmonary edema can occur, and ventilatory compliance can increase. When right atrial pressures exceed left atrial pressures, there can be occurrence of a paradoxical air embolus through a probe-patent foramen ovale. DIC is not a known complication of venous air emboli.

329. **The answer is C (2, 4).** (Stoelting, *Anesthesia and Co-Existing Disease,* 3/e. pp 226–227.) Autonomic hyperreflexia occurs in 65 to 85 percent of patients with lesions above level T7. Regional anesthesia blocks afferent pathways between the stimulus and the spinal cord and thus prevents the response. Beta blockers can produce unopposed alpha agonism with worsened hypertension. Alpha blockers and vasodilators are the agents that should be employed. Bradycardia and hypertension are the major hallmarks. A massive sympathetic and parasympathetic discharge occurs. Parasympathetic tone produces bradycardia but is ineffective in blunting sympathetically induced hypertension.

330. **The answer is A (1, 2, 3).** (Stoelting, *Anesthesia and Co-Existing Disease,* 3/e. pp 226–227.) Loss of sympathetic tone caused by spinal shock leads to unopposed parasympathetic tone; stimulation of the trachea can cause an exaggerated vagal response. Autonomic hyperreflexia usually does not occur until approximately 6 weeks after an injury. Poikilothermy is a feature of early spinal cord injury. Succinylcholine should not be given after the first day after an injury because of the risk of malignant hyperkalemia.

331. **The answer is B (1, 3).** (Stoelting, *Anesthesia and Co-Existing Disease,* 3/e. pp 226–227.) Hypertension and bradycardia in a patient with a spinal cord transection (usually above T8–T10) who receives some kind of stress, such as Foley catheterization, are the hallmarks of autonomic hyperreflexia. With spinal cord transection, there is no central mediation of the sympathetic nervous system below the lesion. With stimulation, there is massive sympathetic outflow from below the lesion. This leads to vascular constriction, which in turn leads to acute hypertension. Above the lesion there is compensatory vasodilation with subsequent nasal stuffiness and flushing, but this is usually not enough to counteract the hypertension. Heart rate slows because of baroreceptor reflexes. Complications include left ventricular dysfunction and cerebral hemorrhage.

332. **The answer is B (1, 3).** (Stoelting, *Anesthesia and Co-Existing Disease,* 3/e. pp 228–230.) Chronic renal failure is a major cause of morbidity in patients who have spinal cord transections. As a result, these patients present repeatedly for GU procedures. The procedures cause a great amount of stimulation, and a full anesthetic must be given to these patients. Adequate anesthesia is needed to prevent sympathetic discharge from below the spinal cord lesion, such as that provided by general, spinal, and less often epidural anesthesia. Local anesthesia is inadequate.

333. **The answer is E (all).** (Miller, 4/e. pp 1327–1329.) Hyperventilation to low CO_2 levels increases EEG activity, and at exceedingly low levels, seizure activity may be evident. Hypercarbia will slow EEG activity and at exceedingly high levels will cause burst suppression. This pattern is not unlike what occurs with increasing concentrations of isoflurane or halothane. Hypoxia causes generalized slowing on the EEG. It is true that hypotension must be significant before changes are seen on EEG, especially if the hypotension is gradual.

334. **The answer is B (1, 3).** (Stoelting, *Anesthesia and Co-Existing Disease,* 3/e. pp 521–522.) The therapeutic mechanism of action of ECT is unknown. However, it is thought that the elicitation of a grand mal seizure that lasts 25 to 60 s is of benefit. Seizure is best documented by EEG monitoring. It also may be followed by isolating one limb from the circulation via a tourniquet before a muscle relaxant is given and watching muscle movement in that limb. Neither the voltage applied nor memory loss is of use in determining the efficacy of ECT.

335. **The answer is B (1, 3).** (Stoelting, *Anesthesia and Co-Existing Disease,* 3/e. pp 521–523.) Loss of bladder and bowel control and post-ECT ileus are not side effects of ECT. With ECT there is a temporal sequence in relation to stimulation of the autonomic nervous system. First there is stimulation of the parasympathetic nervous system. This can last approximately 60 s and may result in bradycardia, hypotension, and increased salivation. After this, there is stimulation of the sympathetic nervous system, which may result in tachycardia, hypertension, and even ventricular premature beats.

336. **The answer is D (4).** (Stoelting, *Anesthesia and Co-Existing Disease,* 3/e. pp 521–523.) ECT can be used safely in patients with orthopedic prostheses, patients who have had heart transplantation, and those who have pacemakers. If ECT is to be used in a patient with a pacemaker, one must know what type of pacemaker it is, why it was put in, and whether it is working before starting ECT therapy. If the pacemaker can be put into the asynchronous mode by a magnet, a magnet should be available. A grand mal seizure can cause an increase in cerebral blood flow and cerebral metabolic rate by as much as seven times. This can lead to an increase in ICP. Therefore, ECT is contraindicated in patients with known increased ICP.

337. **The answer is D (4).** (Stoelting, *Anesthesia and Co-Existing Disease,* 3/e. pp 521–523.) ECT is indicated as therapy in patients who have severe mental depression that is refractory to pharmacologic agents. Although the mechanism of action of ECT is unknown, there is a 75 to 88 percent positive response rate in this group of patients. ECT also has been used in acutely suicidal patients.

338. **The answer is D (4).** (Miller, 4/e. pp 1909–1912.) Morphine and valium can be administered safely so long as respiratory depression and increased P_{CO_2} do not occur. Isoflurane decreases cerebral metabolism and increases cerebral blood flow, causing a net increase in intracranial pressure. Hyperventilation to hypocapnia along with the induction of isoflurane will prevent the increase in ICP that is normally observed in normocapnic patients.

339. **The answer is D (4).** (Miller, 4/e. pp 709–710.) Halothane decreases CSF secretion; enflurane increases CSF secretion. Isoflurane and ketamine have no effect on CSF production.

LIVER AND KIDNEYS

Directions: Each question below contains five suggested responses. Select the **one best** response to each question.

340. Hormonal changes that occur during surgical stimulation and that may have an effect on renal blood flow include increased levels of all the following EXCEPT

    (A)   sympathetic nervous system activity
    (B)   insulin secretion
    (C)   antidiuretic hormone (ADH)
    (D)   renin
    (E)   angiotensin

341. Characteristic changes in patients with end-stage renal disease (ESRD) include all the following EXCEPT

    (A)   a shift to the right of the oxyhemoglobin dissociation curve
    (B)   a decrease in metabolic rate
    (C)   platelet dysfunction
    (D)   anemia
    (E)   increased cardiac output

342. Anesthetic options for extracorporeal shock wave lithotripsy (ESWL) include all the following EXCEPT

    (A)   general anesthesia
    (B)   spinal anesthesia
    (C)   epidural anesthesia
    (D)   local anesthesia
    (E)   intravenous sedation

343. All the following are sequelae of water intoxication induced during transurethral resection of the prostate (TURP) EXCEPT

    (A)   hyponatremia that may lead to cerebral edema
    (B)   central nervous system symptoms including drowsiness, irritability, confusion, and seizures
    (C)   ammonia toxicity leading to eighth cranial nerve (CN VIII) damage
    (D)   pulmonary edema
    (E)   glycine and ammonia toxicity that may lead to transient blindness and a form of encephalopathy

344. Potential benefits of regional anesthesia (epidural, spinal) for transurethral resection of the prostate (TURP) include all the following EXCEPT

    (A)   it may cause better relaxation of urethral musculature and allow easier passage of the resectoscope than general anesthesia

    (B)   an awake patient may demonstrate early signs of water intoxication

    (C)   an awake patient may be able to describe signs of bladder perforation

    (D)   an awake patient may be able to describe signs of bladder overfilling

    (E)   less blood loss will occur during the procedure than occurs with general anesthesia

345. All the following statements are true EXCEPT

    (A)   the liver receives approximately 30 percent of cardiac output

    (B)   the hepatic artery supplies 45 to 50 percent of hepatic oxygen

    (C)   hepatic oxygen delivery is better maintained with isoflurane than with halothane

    (D)   decrease in portal vein blood flow usually is associated with a concomitant decrease in hepatic arterial blood flow

    (E)   local release of vasoconstrictors may decrease hepatic blood flow during abdominal surgery

346. A true statement about hepatic metabolic function is

    (A)   the normal amount of glycogen stored in the liver is depleted after 12 h of starvation

    (B)   normal liver production of 30 g of albumin per day keeps plasma levels of albumin at about 3.5 to 5.5 g/dL

    (C)   acute liver failure rapidly depletes plasma albumin

    (D)   clotting factors produced by the liver include fibrinogen, prothrombin, and factors V, VII, IX, and X

    (E)   decreased plasma binding of drugs is significant at albumin levels less than 5 g/dL

347. Prerenal oliguria can be characterized by

    (A)   urinary sodium > 40 meq/L and urine osmolarity < 250 mosm/L

    (B)   urinary sodium < 40 meq/L and a high urinary potassium level

    (C)   urinary sodium > 40 meq/L and urine osmolarity > 400 mosm/L

    (D)   urinary sodium < 40 meq/L and urinary osmolarity > 400 mosm/L

    (E)   none of the above

Directions: Each question below contains four suggested responses of which **one or more** is correct. Select

(A)	if	**1, 2, and 3**	are correct
(B)	if	**1 and 3**	are correct
(C)	if	**2 and 4**	are correct
(D)	if	**4**	is correct
(E)	if	**1, 2, 3, and 4**	are correct

348. During transurethral resection of the prostate (TURP) for benign prostatic hypertrophy (BPH), the factors that will influence absorption of irrigating solution include the

(1) number of large venous sinuses opened during resection
(2) height of the irrigating solution above the right atrium
(3) length of time of resection
(4) type of irrigating solution

349. The types of irrigating solutions used for transurethral resection of the prostate (TURP) include

(1) 1.5% glycine
(2) normal saline (0.9% NaCl)
(3) Cytol (mannitol and sorbitol)
(4) sterile water

350. Hemodynamic changes that may occur during extracorporeal shock wave lithotripsy (ESWL) include

(1) pooling of blood in the periphery with resultant hypotension
(2) pulmonary edema and congestive heart failure
(3) cardiac dysrhythmias
(4) pacemaker dysfunction

351. True statements about transurethral resection of the prostate (TURP) include

(1) although rare, transient visual disturbances are a potential complication of this procedure
(2) management of severe hyponatremia involves administration of normal or hypertonic saline with a diuretic to prevent circulatory overload
(3) headache, restlessness, or shoulder pain in a patient undergoing TURP may signify some underlying life-threatening process and should be investigated further
(4) metabolism of glycine ammonia may produce postoperative somnolence

352. Major causes of the coagulopathy of chronic renal failure include

(1) decreased concentration of von Willebrand's factor
(2) liver dysfunction
(3) thrombocytopenia
(4) platelet dysfunction

353. True statements with respect to the development of dye-induced acute renal failure include which of the following?

(1) Diabetic patients have an increased risk

(2) Hydration, furosemide, and mannitol have proved effective in reducing the risk

(3) It is usually a self-limiting disease with improvement in 3 to 7 days, but 25 to 50 percent of patients with preexisting renal disease may require dialysis

(4) The complication develops in over 5 percent of patients with normal renal function

354. True statements about kidneys include

(1) blood urea nitrogen (BUN) is an unreliable measure of renal function

(2) changes in serum creatinine are early markers of renal dysfunction

(3) in the elderly, urine specific gravity is an unreliable test of function

(4) decreasing renal perfusion prevents the normal kidney from retaining sodium

355. True statements about renal physiology include which of the following?

(1) During severe hemorrhage or hypoxia, renal blood flow and glomerular filtration rate are well maintained by autoregulation of the renal circulation

(2) Endogenously secreted dopamine is the most important modulator of renal blood flow via its effects on dopamine receptors in the renal vascular bed

(3) Most of the oxygen used by the kidney goes toward maintenance of a normal glomerular filtration rate

(4) Angiotensin produces vasoconstriction, aldosterone release, and sodium retention

356. True statements about renal disease include

(1) hemodialysis improves fluid overload, acidosis, hyperkalemia, and platelet dysfunction

(2) serum electrolyte abnormalities that occur in patients with renal failure include hypercalcemia

(3) serum creatinine is not elevated until approximately 50 percent of renal function is lost

(4) thiopental metabolism is decreased in renal failure

357. Correct descriptions of total body water (TBW) include that it

(1) is distributed relatively more to fat than to lean tissue

(2) is relatively greater in women than in men

(3) composes approximately 40 percent of total body mass through life

(4) declines with age

358. True statements about perioperative oliguria include

    (1)   it is defined as urine output less than 0.5 ml/kg/h

    (2)   it can lead to acute renal failure with a mortality of 50 percent

    (3)   prerenal causes show conservation of tubular function with sodium retention

    (4)   the most common cause of acute renal function perioperatively is renal hypoperfusion

359. True statements about renal transplantation include

    (1)   diseases commonly associated with end-stage renal disease (ESRD) are diabetes mellitus and hypertension

    (2)   cadaveric kidneys can be preserved for 48 to 72 h with low temperature perfusates

    (3)   ABO and human leukocyte antigens are matched between recipient and donor

    (4)   vascular supply to the transplanted kidney comes directly from the aorta

SUMMARY OF DIRECTIONS

A	B	C	D	E
1,2,3	1,3	2,4	4	All are
only	only	only	only	correct

360. Anesthetic management of renal transplantation should consider

    (1) fluoride toxicity from enflurane and sevoflurane, which may be enhanced in the immediate transplant period
    (2) CVP monitoring for fluid management in the perioperative period
    (3) delayed graft rejection, manifest as fever and decreased urine output
    (4) clearance of muscle relaxants, as a newly transplanted functioning kidney does not clear drugs well

361. Replacement of fluid deficits with crystalloid solutions

    (1) should always be isotonic
    (2) have a half-life in the plasma of 15 to 30 min
    (3) can be infused rapidly even if the deficits are greater than 20 percent of blood volume
    (4) is rapidly redistributed to the extravascular space

362. Hypocalcemia in the perioperative period can be due to

    (1) parathyroid hormone deficiency
    (2) transfusion of noncitrated blood
    (3) hyperventilation
    (4) hypophosphatemia

363. In anesthetizing patients with severe hypercalcemia,

    (1) one should avoid drugs metabolized by the liver
    (2) hyperventilation affects the levels of total body calcium
    (3) the response to muscle relaxants is not altered
    (4) adequate hydration is the first line of therapy

364. True statements about magnesium include

    (1) hypermagnesemia is manifested by seizures of hyperreflexia
    (2) hypomagnesemia is manifested by complete heart block on ECG
    (3) low levels of magnesium potentiate narcotics and thiopental
    (4) high levels of magnesium potentiate succinylcholine and curare

365. Hyponatremia or hypernatremia

    (1) is often heralded by subtle changes in mental status
    (2) should be evaluated with regard to total body water content
    (3) is commonly iatrogenic
    (4) should be reversed rapidly to prevent central nervous system dysfunction

366. Treatment of hyponatremia includes

    (1) restriction of water intake
    (2) diuresis
    (3) resuscitation with hypertonic fluid
    (4) demeclocycline

367. True statements about potassium include

(1) hypokalemia is caused by chronic laxative use

(2) decreased mineralocorticoids will cause hypokalemia

(3) hyperkalemia will reduce membrane resting potential, which is shown on ECG as a widened QRS

(4) hyperkalemia will cause U waves on the ECG

368. Side effects of sodium bicarbonate administration include

(1) hypernatremia

(2) increased plasma osmolality

(3) hypokalemia

(4) hypocapnia

369. True statements regarding pH stat acid-base management include

(1) it requires correction of P_{CO_2} to maintain pH at 7.4 at the patient's body temperature

(2) it maintains blood pH of 7.4 independent of the patient's hemoglobin concentration

(3) pH stat behavior is found in hibernating mammals

(4) pH stat behavior is found in ectotherms

370. True statements about the effects of metabolic acidosis on the body include

(1) myocardial contractility is depressed

(2) blood vessels are more responsive to vasoconstrictive drugs

(3) there is an increased risk of ventricular fibrillation

(4) bronchioles are more responsive to bronchodilating drugs

371. Regarding body temperature and its effect on blood gas measurements,

(1) hibernating mammals use pH-stat acid-base regulation at reduced body temperatures

(2) during hypothermic cardiopulmonary bypass, a patient whose blood gases are regulated by the alpha-stat approach will be alkalotic and hypocarbic

(3) rectal or urinary bladder temperatures are valid measurements of central temperature

(4) the pH-stat may be preferable to the alpha-stat approach to blood gas regulation during hypothermic cardiopulmonary bypass because maintenance of a normal pH ensures normal oxygen-hemoglobin affinity and normal oxygen delivery to the tissues

372. Alpha stat acid-base management

(1) is associated with loss of cerebral blood flow autoregulation during hypothermia and high P_{CO_2}

(2) is associated with a higher cardiac index and myocardial contractility during hypothermia

(3) is associated with a higher incidence of ventricular fibrillation during hypothermia

(4) may be associated with lower cerebral blood flow during hypothermia

373. Metabolic acidosis with an elevated anion gap occurs in patients with

  (1)   excessive GI losses
  (2)   inhibition of carbonic anhydrase
  (3)   renal tubular acidosis
  (4)   diabetic ketoacidosis

374. A patient has been diagnosed as having metabolic acidosis with ventilatory compensation. Blood gas measurements that support this diagnosis include

  (1)   pH 7.4, P_{CO_2} 30, HCO_3 16 mM/L
  (2)   pH 7.20, P_{CO_2} 43, HCO_3 30 mM/L
  (3)   pH 7.42, P_{CO_2} 40, HCO_3 26 mM/L
  (4)   pH 7.30, P_{CO_2} 30, HCO_3 14 mM/L

375. A rightward shift in the oxyhemoglobin dissociation curve is caused by

  (1)   elevated body temperature
  (2)   fetal hemoglobin
  (3)   elevated P_{CO_2}
  (4)   decreased 2,3-DPG

376. If a Swan-Ganz catheter is inserted into a patient with alcoholic cirrhosis, which of the following scenarios may be seen?

  (1)   High cardiac output and low systemic vascular resistance (SVR)
  (2)   Low filling pressures and a high cardiac output
  (3)   High filling pressures and a low cardiac output
  (4)   High cardiac output and high SVR

SUMMARY OF DIRECTIONS

A	B	C	D	E
1,2,3	1,3	2,4	4	All are
only	only	only	only	correct

377. Perioperative risk in patients with liver disease can be assessed by looking at

(1) bilirubin level
(2) degree of ascites
(3) albumin level
(4) white blood cell count

378. Hepatic blood flow is decreased by

(1) isoflurane
(2) cholecystectomy
(3) halothane
(4) spinal anesthesia

LIVER AND KIDNEYS

A N S W E R S

340. **The answer is B.** (Stoelting, *Anesthesia and Co-Existing Disease,* 3/e. pp 289–290.) Insulin secretion does not increase during surgical stimulation, and insulin levels do not have any effect on renal blood flow. The kidney is innervated by the sympathetic nervous system. Catecholamine levels, which do increase with surgical stimulation, may increase renal vascular resistance and therefore decrease renal blood flow. Other hormonal changes that occur during surgical stimulation are increases in ADH, renin, and angiotensin, which also decrease renal blood flow. It should be noted that preoperative hydration will attenuate these hormonal changes and maintain renal blood flow.

341. **The answer is B.** (Stoelting, *Anesthesia and Co-Existing Disease,* 3/e. p 297.) Metabolic rate in ESRD does not change because of the disease process. A major consideration during anesthetic management with ESRD is preservation of the compensatory responses to chronic anemia. Cardiac output must be maintained by keeping right heart filling pressures at steady state and by preserving myocardial contractility.

342. **The answer is E.** (Stoelting, *Anesthesia and Co-Existing Disease,* 3/e. p 438.) ESWL is extremely painful, and a patient will not be able to tolerate the procedure under intravenous sedation alone. Local anesthesia is adequate if it is done carefully and correctly. Local anesthesia consists of a liberal field block in the region where the lithotriptor will be aimed. Intercostal nerve blocks at the eleventh and twelfth ribs also are useful.

343. **The answer is C.** (Stoelting, *Anesthesia and Co-Existing Disease,* 3/e. pp 308–309.) Glycine is an amino acid that is metabolized in the liver by the urea cycle; one of the by-products is ammonia. Ammonia can pass the blood-brain barrier and cause drowsiness and a form of encephalopathy. Serum ammonia levels may be helpful in determining whether encephalopathy is occurring. It is believed that glycine can cross the blood-brain barrier and act as a false neurotransmitter that causes visual disturbances but not eighth cranial nerve (CN VIII) damage.

344. **The answer is A.** (Stoelting, *Anesthesia and Co-Existing Disease*, 3/e. pp 308–309.) Urethral musculature is relaxed equally with regional anesthesia and general anesthesia. Regional anesthesia may lead to less blood loss, as it does in other types of procedures. There are many benefits to having an awake patient who is receiving a TURP. One of the early signs of water intoxication is an early onset of mental confusion. Perforation of the bladder will lead to the patient's complaining of subdiaphragmatic pain. Also, if the bladder is perforated, when the abdomen is examined under regional anesthesia, it will feel rigid as opposed to the usual relaxed state. Some older resectoscopes do not allow for irrigation drainage and must be removed periodically. The symptoms of an overfilled bladder are similar to those of perforation.

345. **The answer is D.** (Stoelting, *Anesthesia and Co-Existing Disease*, 3/e. p 253.) Decreased portal vein blood flow usually is associated with an increase in hepatic arterial blood flow. This increase in hepatic arterial blood flow is considered an attempt to maintain oxygen supply and clearance of exogenous and endogenous compounds with a high hepatic extraction. Halothane interferes with this balance, while isoflurane does not.

346. **The answer is D.** (Stoelting, *Anesthesia and Co-Existing Disease*, 3/e. p 251.) Enough glycogen is stored in the liver to last for 24 to 48 h of starvation. The liver normally produces 10 to 15 g of albumin daily to maintain the normal range of 3.5 to 5.5 g/dL. Plasma binding of drugs is not seriously affected until levels fall to 2.5 g/dL. Albumin has a half-life of 14 to 21 days in plasma, making it unlikely that acute liver failure will affect drug binding.

347. **The answer is D.** (Stoelting, *Anesthesia and Co-Existing Disease*, 3/e. p 303.) With prerenal oliguria, the kidney is attempting to conserve sodium and intravascular fluid. Glomerular filtration rate and renal cortical blood flow have not diminished at this point. As a result, the kidney is still able to reabsorb fluid and concentrate urine. Urinary sodium levels will be below 40 meq/L, and urine osmolarity will be above 400 mosm/L.

348. **The answer is A (1, 2, 3).** (Stoelting, *Anesthesia and Co-Existing Disease*, 3/e. pp 308–309.) The type of irrigating solution used is not a determinant of fluid absorption during a TURP. It is very difficult to ascertain how much irrigating solution will be absorbed during the procedure. Estimates vary from approximately 10 to 30 mL/min of resection time. It also seems that when resection time is greater than 1 h, there is a greater risk of fluid absorption. A short resection time does not provide a guarantee against massive fluid absorption, but it may be less likely to occur. There have been many reports of fluid overload, congestive heart failure, and water intoxication in cases with resection times of 5 to 10 min.

349. **The answer is B (1, 3).** (Stoelting, *Anesthesia and Co-Existing Disease,* 3/e. pp 308–309.) Normal saline (0.9% NaCl) will cause no danger to the patient if it is absorbed via the prostatic venous sinuses because it has the same osmolarity as blood. It is not used because it will cause a dispersion of the electrical charge during electrocoagulation. Sterile water is not used because when it is absorbed, swelling and then lysis of red blood cells will occur because of its low osmolarity. Although Cytol is used, it acts as an excellent medium for bacterial proliferation, which can lead to urosepsis.

350. **The answer is E (all).** (Stoelting, *Anesthesia and Co-Existing Disease,* 3/e. pp 307–308.) Even though the patient is in the sitting position, which causes pooling of blood in the periphery and possibly leads to hypotension, immersion in water may increase hydrostatic pressure and lead to increased venous return to the right heart and concomitant congestive heart failure. Shock waves from the lithotriptor are timed with the patient's ECG to occur during the absolute refractory period to prevent dysrhythmias. If the patient has an inhibitory type of pacemaker, a shock wave can be sensed and may lead to pacemaker dysfunction.

351. **The answer is E (all).** (Stoelting, *Anesthesia and Co-Existing Disease,* 3/e. pp 308–309.) Transient blindness is a rare but reported complication after TURP. This is thought to be due to glycine toxicity and may occur when large volumes of glycine solutions are absorbed. Headache, restlessness, and shoulder pain must prompt careful evaluation for possible TURP syndrome; they may otherwise evolve to seizures and even death. The surgeon should complete the procedure as soon as possible.

352. **The answer is D (4).** (Stoelting, *Anesthesia and Co-Existing Disease,* 3/e. pp 297–298.) A major cause of coagulopathy in chronic renal failure is platelet dysfunction, i.e., decreased platelet adhesiveness caused by uremia. A convenient measure of this type of platelet dysfunction is an elevated bleeding time. Platelet number is usually normal. The treatment of platelet dysfunction consists of dialysis. Systemic heparinization, which is needed in dialysis, is another cause of coagulopathy. Decreased concentrations of von Willebrand's factor and liver dysfunction are minor factors that may contribute to coagulopathy.

353. **The answer is A (1, 2, 3).** (Miller, 4/e. pp 1172–1173.) Diabetic patients have an increased risk, but those with normal renal function have a minimal risk. The complication develops in approximately 2 percent of patients with normal renal function. Hydration and the use of furosemide and mannitol are effective in reducing the risk of dye-induced acute renal failure.

354. **The answer is B (1, 3).** (Miller, 4/e. pp 1304–1305.) BUN is freely filtered at the glomerulus but is partially reabsorbed in the renal tubules. Reabsorption is enhanced by dehydration, which elevates BUN. BUN also is elevated by a high-protein diet, gastrointestinal bleeding, and accelerated metabolism (sepsis, for example). Elevations of creatinine and BUN are both late signs of renal dysfunction because of the large GFR reserve. In the elderly, renal water concentration is normally slightly impaired, making specific gravity an unreliable test in this group. Decreasing renal perfusion actually stimulates normal kidneys to retain and conserve sodium and water.

355. **The answer is D (4).** (Miller, 4/e. pp 665, 677–683.) Under extreme conditions or during infusions of high concentrations of norepinephrine or epinephrine, renal blood flow and glomerular filtration rate fall dramatically. The physiologic role of dopamine in renal hemodynamics is uncertain, but it is not thought to be an important factor most of the time. The kidney expends most of its energy on sodium transport. The stimulus for angiotensin production is renin release by the afferent arterioles of the kidneys. The stimuli for renin release include blood pressure in the afferent arterioles, sodium content of those arterioles, and levels of circulating catecholamines.

356. **The answer is B (1, 3).** (Miller, 4/e. pp 1955–1957.) Hemodialysis also improves uremic encephalopathy and neuropathy. It should be remembered that residual heparinization can last a few hours after hemodialysis; protamine can be used to counteract heparin if needed. Potassium, phosphate, and magnesium are all elevated in renal failure, but calcium is decreased and patients are prone to tetany if they are acutely made alkalotic (as with hyperventilation or bicarbonate therapy). Urinary creatinine clearance will indicate depressed renal function early in renal insufficiency, but it is not until half of renal function is lost that serum urea nitrogen and creatinine start to increase. Patients who have ≤ 50 percent reduction in renal function need not be managed differently from normal patients and have no increased risk with anesthesia. The induction dose of thiopental should be decreased in renal failure, but the reason is that more free drug is available as a result of decreased binding to albumin and, under acidic conditions, more un-ionized (i.e., active) drug is present. Metabolism of thiopental is unchanged in renal failure, and in any event, redistribution rather than metabolism dictates induction dose.

357. **The answer is D (4).** (Miller, 3/e. pp 1595–1597.) Fat tissue contains less TBW (400 mL/kg) than does lean tissue (650 mL/kg). Women have more fat than men and therefore have less TBW than men. Throughout life TBW constitutes about 60 percent of total body mass. It is highest at birth (75 percent) and gradually declines with age.

358. **The answer is E (all).** (Stoelting, *Anesthesia and Co-Existing Disease*, 3/e. p 303.) It is critically important to promptly diagnose and reverse the causes of oliguria. They can be classified as prerenal, such as hypovolemia; renal, as seen in acute tubular necrosis; and postrenal, usually from ureteral obstruction. Urine sodium values are high in renal causes and low in prerenal causes. Urine osmolarity is high in prerenal causes and lower in renal problems.

359. **The answer is B (1, 3).** (Stoelting, *Anesthesia and Co-Existing Disease,* 3/e. p 310.) Other diseases associated with ESRD are glomerulonephritis and polycystic kidney disease. Cadaveric kidneys can be preserved for only 24 to 36 h. Vascular supply to the new graft comes from the iliac vessels.

360. **The answer is A (1, 2, 3).** (Stoelting, *Anesthesia and Co-Existing Disease*, 3/e. pp 310–311.) Clearance of fluoride ions is dependent upon GFR, which may be decreased in the immediate transplant period. Assuming there is no significant heart disease, CVP monitoring should give adequate assessment of fluid status. A newly transplanted functioning kidney clears drugs as well as normal kidneys do.

361. **The answer is C (2, 4).** (Miller, 4/e. pp 1607–1611.) Fluid deficits should be replaced by the type of fluid that is lost. Perspiration and insensible losses tend to be hypotonic, while intestinal losses vary in ionicity depending on the site of fluid loss. Replacements can be rapidly infused preoperatively or early in the surgery if the deficit is small. Large deficits (greater than 20 percent of blood volume) should be infused more slowly and before surgery if possible. Most crystalloid infusions will be distributed between the interstitial space and the plasma at a ratio of 3:1. This will occur over 15 to 30 min.

362. **The answer is B (1, 3).** (Stoelting, *Anesthesia and Co-Existing Disease,* 3/e. pp 330–331.) Parathyroid hormone regulates bone reabsorption and inhibits renal excretion of calcium. If the parathyroid glands are removed, as occurs during thyroid surgery, an acute decrease in calcium manifested by hypotension, muscle cramps, laryngospasm, and dysrhythmias occurs. Emergency treatment consists of calcium chloride 15 mg/kg or calcium gluconate 45 mg/kg IV. Citrate in banked blood products binds calcium. This will cause hypocalcemia when the transfusion rate exceeds 1 unit per 5 min. Noncitrated blood does not bind calcium and therefore does not affect calcium concentrations. Hyperventilation causes respiratory alkalosis and can lead to binding of calcium by proteins. This results in reduced ionized calcium concentrations and causes hypotension. Bicarbonate therapy, by causing a metabolic alkalosis, can have the same effect. Hyperphosphatemia increases tissue deposition of calcium and causes hypocalcemia.

363. **The answer is D (4).** (Stoelting, *Anesthesia and Co-Existing Disease,* 3/e. p 330.) Hypercalcemia can cause impairment in urine-concentrating abilities and even renal failure. If renal failure is present, drugs dependent on renal metabolism and excretion should be avoided. The liver is unaffected in hypercalcemia. Hypercalcemia may cause skeletal muscle weaknesses, and so muscle relaxants can be potentiated. Adequate hydration with saline solutions is the first line of therapy for hypercalcemia. This dilutes plasma levels of calcium and inhibits renal reabsorption of calcium.

364. **The answer is D (4).** (Miller, 4/e. pp 1604–1605. Stoelting, *Anesthesia and Co-Existing Disease,* 2/e. p 468.) Magnesium is involved in membrane excitability. Neuromuscular depression occurs with high levels of magnesium. Though low magnesium levels can widen the QRS and cause peaked T waves, heart block is caused by high levels of magnesium. Magnesium levels do not interact with anesthetic drugs other than the muscle relaxants. With high levels of magnesium, one gets a potentiation of depolarizing and nondepolarizing muscle relaxants.

365. **The answer is A (1, 2, 3).** (Miller, 4/e. pp 1602–1603.) Sodium does not cross the blood-brain barrier, although water does. Therefore, hypernatremia results in cerebral shrinkage, while hyponatremia may result in cerebral edema. Both situations can cause changes in mental status. Hyponatremia most commonly is due to hypervolemia, and hypernatremia usually is due to hypovolemia. Assessment of volume status often yields the etiology of the sodium disturbance. Hyponatremia can occur with excessive water absorption, as in TURP surgery, and with overhydration. Sodium deficiency can be caused by diuretics and inadequate replacement. Iatrogenic causes of hypernatremia include water deprivation, sodium load from certain antibiotics and sodium bicarbonate, and excess saline administration. Sodium imbalances should be treated slowly to prevent nervous system dysfunction.

366. **The answer is E (all).** (Miller, 4/e. pp 973–974.) When hyponatremia is due to hypervolemia, restriction of water intake is the primary treatment. Diuretics, such as furosemide, can aid in excretion of excess water and restore normal serum sodium concentrations. When there are CNS signs—such as confusion, seizures, and coma—slow infusions of hypertonic saline solutions (3 to 5%) can restore normal sodium concentrations. If hyponatremia is due to the inappropriate secretion of antidiuretic hormone (ADH), treatment should include demeclocycline. This drug interferes with the ability of renal tubules to concentrate urine; the dilute urine can then reverse the hyponatremia.

367. **The answer is B (1, 3).** (Miller, 4/e. pp 974–976.) Inadequate intake and excess GI losses such as from diarrhea, chronic use of laxatives, and nasogastric suctioning are causes of hypokalemia. Aldosterone is the primary mineralocorticoid. It causes reabsorption of sodium at the expense of potassium and hydrogen ions. Therefore, an excess of mineralocorticoids will cause hypokalemia. With hyperkalemia, the QRS will merge with the T wave and create a sine wave on ECG. U waves are signs of hypokalemia.

368. **The answer is A (1, 2, 3).** (Miller, 4/e. pp 1395–1396.) Sodium bicarbonate has a very high osmolarity and sodium content, which can be detrimental to certain patients with CHF. In patients who are acidotic and hypocalemic, alkalinization can further worsen hypokalemia. The breakdown of sodium bicarbonate by the body produces carbon dioxide, which can result in hypercapnia and a paradoxical respiratory acidosis unless ventilation is increased.

369. **The answer is B (1, 3).** (Miller, 4/e. pp 1397–1398.) The pH stat measurements are dependent on the patient's temperature and assume normal hemoglobin levels. Measurements usually are made with electrodes at 37°C. Since the P_{CO_2} of blood decreases with cooling, CO_2 is added to the measured sample to approximate patient conditions. Alpha stat behavior is found in ectotherms.

370. **The answer is B (1, 3).** (Miller, 4/e. pp 1393–1397.) Excessive hydrogen ion concentrations have a depressant effect on the body and interfere with enzyme activity. Blood vessels tend to vasodilate and be unresponsive to vasoconstrictive drugs. Contractivity is depressed, as is the ventricular fibrillation threshold. Bronchodilators such as isoproterenol also have an attenuated effect on bronchioles.

371. **The answer is A (1, 2, 3).** (Miller, 4/e. pp 1397–1398.) In hibernating mammals acid-base status is adjusted as body temperature declines so that a pH of 7.4 is maintained regardless of body temperature. With the alpha-stat approach, the blood gas is uncorrected for temperature. Rectal and urinary bladder temperatures are valid; however, during rapid rewarming, these temperatures lag behind those of other sites for measuring central temperatures, e.g., the pulmonary artery, esophagus, and tympanic membrane. The effect of maintaining a normal pH will be offset by the effect of hypothermia with regard to oxygen-hemoglobin affinity. In addition, metabolic rate is markedly reduced during hypothermia, and this limits the impact of a left-shifted oxyhemoglobin dissociation curve.

372. **The answer is C (2, 4).** (Miller, 4/e. pp 1397–1398.) Cerebral flow autoregulation during hypothermia and with high P_{CO_2} is better preserved with alpha stat than with pH stat. A lower incidence of ventricular fibrillation is found during hypothermia with alpha stat management.

373. **The answer is D (4).** (Miller, 4/e. pp 1393–1397.) The anion gap, $Na^+ - (Cl^- + CO_2$ content), is a measure of excess metabolic acid production or a decrease in its excretion. Changes in bicarbonate levels, such as seen in GI losses or with carbonic anhydrase inhibition, do not affect the anion gap; neither does renal tubular acidosis. Only situations that result in excess acid production, such as diabetic ketoacidosis and lactic acidosis, or decreased acid excretion, such as renal failure, cause a rise in the anion gap.

374. **The answer is D (4).** (Miller, 4/e. pp 1391–1397.) Ventilation can never compensate completely for a metabolic acidosis. Therefore, the pH will never equal or exceed 7.4. Also, in metabolic acidosis, HCO_3 is less than 24 mM/L. Established nomograms can help with the diagnosis as well. The diagram below shows the six fundamental acid-base states. The

P_{CO_2} = 40 mmHg and 10 sl lines indicate uncompensated states for metabolic and respiratory derangements, respectively. The pH = 7.4 line represents complete compensation.

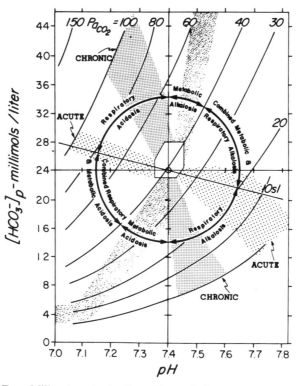

From Miller, *Anesthesia,* 4/e, with permission.

375. **The answer is B (1, 3).** (Miller, 4/e. p 597.) Rightward shift of the oxyhemoglobin dissociation curve is associated with a decreased affinity of hemoglobin for oxygen. Increases in body temperature, P_{CO_2}, and 2,3-DPG as well as decreases in pH and fetal hemoglobin levels will cause a rightward shift in the curve.

376. **The answer is B (1, 3).** (Stoelting, *Anesthesia and Co-Existing Disease,* 3/e. pp 264–265.) With alcoholic cirrhosis, initially one will see signs of a hyperdynamic circulation. With Swan-Ganz catheter monitoring, one will see normal to high filling pressures, high cardiac output, and low systemic vascular resistance. The possible reasons for this include a high intravascular fluid volume, decreased viscosity of blood secondary to anemia, and arteriovenous shunting in the lungs. With end-stage cirrhosis, a dilated cardiomyopathy with biventricular dysfunction develops. With Swan-Ganz monitoring, one will see high filling pressures and low cardiac output, a hypodynamic circulation.

377. **The answer is A (1, 2, 3).** (Stoelting, *Anesthesia and Co-Existing Disease,* 3/e. p 266.) Prothrombin time, encephalopathy, and nutritional status are also factors to assess.

378. **The answer is E (all).** (Stoelting, *Anesthesia and Co-Existing Disease,* 3/e. p 253.) Inhalational agents all decrease hepatic blood flow. The nearer the operative site to the liver, the greater the reduction in hepatic blood flow. Regional anesthesia decreases hepatic blood flow by decreasing perfusion pressure.

HEMATOLOGY

Directions: Each question below contains four suggested responses of which **one or more** is correct. Select

(A)	if	**1, 2, and 3**	are correct
(B)	if	**1 and 3**	are correct
(C)	if	**2 and 4**	are correct
(D)	if	**4**	is correct
(E)	if	**1, 2, 3, and 4**	are correct

379. Autotransfusion of salvaged blood is relatively or absolutely contraindicated from

(1) an infected wound
(2) operative field with tumor cells
(3) operative field with potential contamination by intestinal contents
(4) operative field with blood loss of less than 2 units

380. Contraindications for normovolemic hemodilution include

(1) anemia
(2) coronary artery disease
(3) carotid artery disease
(4) small infants

381. True statements about hemoglobin and oxygen transport include which of the following?

(1) The change in hemoglobin saturation is much greater at a P_{O_2} of 30 mmHg than at a P_{O_2} of 70 mmHg

(2) Fetal hemoglobin is capable of carrying more oxygen at a low P_{O_2} than is normal adult hemoglobin

(3) The Bohr effect facilitates binding of oxygen to hemoglobin in the lungs and release of oxygen from hemoglobin in the tissues

(4) A patient with a hematocrit of 45 percent, a hemoglobin of 15 mg/dL, and a circulating blood volume of 4500 mL can carry a total of approximately 250 mL of oxygen in the blood at any one time

382. A 50-year old woman on coumarin needs emergency surgery. Which of the following would constitute appropriate management for neutralization of coumarin?

(1) Administration of heparin
(2) Administration of vitamin K
(3) Administration of protamine
(4) Transfusion of blood or fresh frozen plasma

383. Correct statements regarding heparin include that it

(1) can easily cross the placenta to the fetus

(2) results in a decrease in antithrombin III activity with continued use

(3) is present endogenously in a high concentration in the kidney

(4) results in mild thrombocytopenia in 40 percent of patients

384. True statements regarding coumarin include that it

(1) works in the liver by interfering with the production of factors II, VII, IX, and X

(2) may be given orally or intravenously

(3) is a known teratogen

(4) is poorly protein-bound in the plasma

385. True hematologic principles include

(1) the concentration of factor VIII in plasma necessary for hemostasis during major surgery is greater than 30 percent of normal

(2) fresh frozen plasma (FFP) is not considered a first line of treatment for hemophilia A

(3) factor VIII concentrates carry a greater risk of being infected with a virus than does cryoprecipitate

(4) the elimination half-time of factor VIII is 18 to 24 h

386. Drugs that are known to precipitate porphyria include

(1) phenytoin
(2) thiopental
(3) diazepam
(4) lidocaine

387. Drugs that are safe in a patient with a history of acute intermittent porphyria include

(1) narcotics
(2) nitrous oxide
(3) droperidol
(4) chlordiazepoxide

388. Citrate intoxication associated with blood transfusion is

(1) unlikely to occur unless citrate phosphate-dextrose (CPD) blood infusion exceeds 150 mL/70 kg per minute
(2) a direct effect of citrate on the vascular smooth muscle with resultant hypotension
(3) related to a decrease in ionized calcium
(4) further aggravated by hypoventilation

389. Blood products that transmit viruses include

(1) fresh frozen plasma
(2) platelets
(3) cryoprecipitate
(4) albumin

390. Regarding stored whole blood,

(1) P-50 increases with length of time stored
(2) plasma pH decreases with length of storage
(3) 2,3-DPG increases with length of storage
(4) metabolic alkalosis frequently follows massive transfusion

391. Regarding transfusion practices, it is appropriate to give

(1) cryoprecipitate from a type AB donor to a type O recipient
(2) packed red cells from a type A donor to a type AB recipient
(3) fresh frozen plasma from a type B donor to a type O recipient
(4) fresh frozen plasma from a type B donor to a type AB recipient

SUMMARY OF DIRECTIONS

A	B	C	D	E
1,2,3 only	1,3 only	2,4 only	4 only	All are correct

392. True statements about platelet dysfunction include which of the following?

(1) The platelet disorder that occurs with massive blood transfusions is due to the detrimental effects of the citrate used in stored blood

(2) Aspirin, through its effect on thromboxane formation, impairs platelet aggregation

(3) Impaired platelet aggregation from a deficiency of factor VIII occurs in sickle cell disease

(4) Platelet dysfunction often occurs with cardiopulmonary bypass and is primarily due to the mechanical disruption of platelets by the heart-lung machine

393. Accurate descriptions of platelets include that they

(1) have a normal life span of 25 to 30 days

(2) must be given according to ABO blood type compatibility

(3) are frozen until ready for use

(4) carry a risk of bacterial contamination

394. With regard to transfusion reactions,

(1) erythema and urticaria constitute evidence of a hemolytic reaction

(2) severity of a hemolytic reaction is positively correlated with the volume of blood infused

(3) complaints of substernal or back pain, dyspnea, and nausea are symptoms of a hemolytic reaction readily apparent to anesthesiologists

(4) shivering secondary to a mild febrile reaction may be treated with meperidine

395. True statements regarding blood transfusions include which of the following?

(1) If a hemolytic transfusion reaction is suspected, it is safe to continue the transfusion as long as steroids and diphenhydramine (Benadryl) are given promptly

(2) A patient with blood type A can safely receive fresh frozen plasma from a donor with blood type A or O

(3) Common intraoperative signs of a hemolytic transfusion reaction include hypertension and ventricular bigeminy

(4) The use of donor-designated blood has not significantly decreased the incidence of infection caused by blood transfusions

396. Regarding acute hemolytic transfusion reactions,

(1) fatal acute hemolytic transfusion reactions are most likely due to ABO incompatibility

(2) when acute hemolytic transfusion reaction is suspected, the transfusion should be stopped immediately to limit the amount of volume transfused

(3) signs of acute hemolytic transfusion reaction under general anesthesia include hypotension, bleeding diathesis, and hemoglobinuria

(4) the most serious reactions involve extravascular hemolysis

397. True statements regarding von Willebrand's disease include that it

(1) is transmitted in an autosomal dominant manner

(2) is due to the absence of a protein necessary for adequate functioning of factor VIII and platelets

(3) is manifested by a decreased plasma concentration of factor VIII among other things

(4) may be treated with either factor VIII concentrates or cryoprecipitate

398. The functions of von Willebrand's factor include

(1) optimal activity of factor IX

(2) optimal activity of factor VIII

(3) prevention of clot lysis

(4) optimal platelet function

399. Accurate descriptions of beta thalassemia include which of the following?

(1) Beta thalassemia normally is not manifested in newborns

(2) Beta thalassemia minor manifests as a mild hypochromic, microcytic anemia

(3) Beta thalassemia intermedia is associated with increased hemoglobin F levels and decreased 2,3-DPG levels

(4) Beta thalassemia major is not compatible with life

400. Correct statements about hemophilia A include that it

(1) is due to diminished factor VIII activity

(2) may result in spontaneous hemorrhage

(3) manifests clinically as hemarthroses, hematuria, and deep tissue bleeding

(4) may be screened for by prothrombin time

401. True statements regarding hemophilia B include

(1) hemophilia B is due to a deficiency of factor IX

(2) clinical features include purpura, petechiae, and epistaxis

(3) partial thromboplastin time is prolonged

(4) fresh frozen plasma is the treatment of choice

402. Anesthetic management of a patient with sickle cell disease should include

(1) maintenance of intravascular fluid volume

(2) prevention of acidosis

(3) optimal oxygenation

(4) exchange transfusions to increase hemoglobin A to 20 percent

403. True statements regarding sickle cell disease include

(1) hemoglobin S has valine substituted for glutamic acid at the sixth position of the beta-hemoglobin chain

(2) persons with sickle cell trait are heterozygous with the hemoglobin genotype AS

(3) the renal medulla is a frequent site of vascular occlusion with sickle cells

(4) formation of sickle cells tends to be greater in arteries than in veins

404. Sickle cell disease and sickle cell trait may be characterized by which of the following statements?

(1) Sickling can occur in patients with sickle cell trait when Pa_{O_2} is at 40 to 50 mmHg

(2) Infection, acidosis, and dehydration can precipitate a sickling crisis in patients with sickle cell disease

(3) The use of Esmarch tourniquets is contraindicated for these patients because a low-flow state to the extremity is produced, which predisposes to local cooling, intravascular stasis, and acidosis

(4) Patients with sickle cell disease have a tendency toward early desaturation

405. True statements regarding methemoglobin include that it

(1) is hemoglobin A where the iron exists in the ferrous rather than ferric form

(2) causes a shift in the oxyhemoglobin dissociation curve to the left

(3) results in cyanosis when plasma levels exceed 5 g/dL

(4) may be increased by treatment with nitrate-containing substances such as sodium nitroprusside and nitroglycerin

HEMATOLOGY

ANSWERS

379. The answer is A (1, 2, 3). (Miller, 4/e. pp 1653–1656.) Although blood salvage of less than 2 units is not considered cost-effective, it is not contraindicated.

380. The answer is A (1, 2, 3). (Miller, 4/e. pp 1651–1653.) Contraindications for normovolemic hemodilution include coronary artery disease, carotid artery disease, hepatic dysfunction, renal insufficiency, and anemia. The technique has been employed successfully in small infants and is not contraindicated in this patient population.

381. The answer is A (1, 2, 3). (Stoelting, *Anesthesia and Coexisting Disease,* 3/e. pp 393–395.) In hypoxic tissues, large amounts of oxygen can be unloaded. Fetal hemoglobin has a higher affinity for oxygen than does adult hemoglobin. The P_{O_2} of blood entering the fetus is 28 mmHg; in the adult, hemoglobin would be 50 percent saturated at this P_{O_2}, but fetal hemoglobin would be 80 percent saturated. Fetal hemoglobin disappears by age 4 to 6 months. In the lungs, transfer of carbon dioxide out of the blood into alveoli renders blood alkalotic; this shifts the oxygen-hemoglobin dissociation curve to the left, which facilitates oxygen binding to hemoglobin. At the tissues, carbon dioxide diffuses into the blood, rendering it acidotic, which shifts the curve to the right and facilitates oxygen release from hemoglobin to the tissues. This carbon dioxide shifting of the curve is known as the *Bohr effect.* Each milligram of hemoglobin can carry 1.34 mL of oxygen when hemoglobin is fully saturated, and so 15 mg/100 mL × 1.34 mL/mg × 4500 mL = 1000 mL. Of interest, by comparison, 4500 mL of blood is capable of carrying only 13.5 mL of dissolved oxygen at a P_{O_2} of 100 mmHg (0.003 mL oxygen per 100 mL blood for each mmHg of P_{O_2}, or 0.003/100 × 100 × 4500 = 13.5 mL).

382. **The answer is C (2, 4).** (Barash, 3/e. pp 210–211.) Coumarin inhibits vitamin K–dependent factors II, VII, IX, and X. Low doses will prolong prothrombin time (PT) but not partial thromboplastin time (PTT) because only factor IX is affected. At higher doses, all factors are affected, resulting in prolongation of PT and PTT. Administration of vitamin K or blood and plasma that contain factors II, VII, IX, and X will neutralize the effect of coumarin.

383. **The answer is C (2, 4).** (Barash, 3/e. p 211.) Heparin is a large, poorly lipid-soluble molecular that, unlike coumarin, does not cross the placenta easily. While heparin works by initially increasing the formation of antithrombin III, which itself decreases thrombin and factor X activity, continued use of heparin results in decreased antithrombin III activity. Heparin is present in a high concentration in the liver as well as in mast cells and basophils. Up to 40 percent of patients treated with heparin experience a clinically insignificant thrombocytopenia. A much smaller percentage experience a more severe thrombocytopenia.

384. **The answer is A (1, 2, 3).** (Stoelting, *Pharmacology and Physiology*, 2/e. pp 472–474.) Coumarin interferes with the production of the vitamin K–dependent factors II, VII, IX, and X. It may be given either orally or intravenously, although the anticoagulant effect takes 8 to 12 h either way. Coumarin is a known teratogen that results in anomalies such as blindness and hypoplasia. It is approximately 97 percent bound to albumin.

385. **The answer is A (1, 2, 3).** (Stoelting, *Anesthesia and Co-Existing Disease,* 3/e. pp 411–412, 599, 600.) Greater than 30 percent of normal plasma concentrations of factor VIII are thought to be necessary for hemostasis for major surgery. FFP is not a first-line therapy for hemophilia A. Factor VIII concentrates and cryoprecipitate are more specific and necessitate less volume infusion. Factor VIII concentrates are more expensive and create an increased risk of viral contamination as they are prepared from pooled plasma, whereas cryoprecipitate comes from a single donor. The elimination half-time of factor VIII is 10 to 12 h.

386. **The answer is E (all).** (Stoelting, *Anesthesia and Co-Existing Disease,* 3/e. pp 375–378.) Barbiturates, benzodiazepines, hydantoin anticonvulsants, and lidocaine can all induce porphyria. Porphyrias are genetic disorders involving defects in heme synthesis. Their symptoms include abdominal pain and neurologic symptoms; many also have cutaneous manifestations.

387. **The answer is A (1, 2, 3).** (Stoelting, *Anesthesia and Co-Existing Disease,* 3/e. pp 375–378.) The first three listed drugs are considered safe in patients with acute intermittent porphyria. Drugs such as chlordiazepoxide induce δ-aminolevulinic acid (ALA) synthetase, which exacerbates the symptoms of porphyria. Symptoms include colicky pain, nausea, and psychiatric disorders.

388. **The answer is B (1, 3).** (Miller, 4/e. p 1631.) There is no direct effect of citrate on the vascular smooth muscle. Hypotension is secondary to citrate binding of calcium. Citrate metabolism is dependent on the liver; therefore, it is further aggravated by liver disease. In addition, hypothermia and hyperventilation can increase the possibility of citrate intoxication.

389. **The answer is A (1, 2, 3).** (Stoelting, *Anesthesia and Co-Existing Disease,* 3/e. p 421.) Albumin solutions are heated to 60°C for an extended period, so that even though albumin comes from pooled donors, viruses are killed in the sterilization process.

390. **The answer is C (2, 4).** (Stoelting, *Anesthesia and Co-Existing Disease,* 3/e. pp 422–425.) P-50 on the oxyhemoglobin dissociation curve decreases as storage time of whole blood increases. Plasma pH decreases over time in stored whole blood. 2,3-DPG decreases with length of storage. Metabolic alkalosis more frequently occurs after massive transfusions than does metabolic acidosis. This is thought to be secondary to the conversion of citrate to bicarbonate.

391. **The answer is A (1, 2, 3).** (Miller, 4/e. pp 1620–1622.) Remember, cryoprecipitate is a plasma product that contains few if any red blood cells. Since the donor's blood type is AB, the donor's plasma contains no anti-A or anti-B antibodies. This makes an AB donor the "universal donor" for plasma products. The AB recipient contains no anti-A or anti-B antibodies; therefore, infusion of type A red cells is acceptable. Type B donor plasma (e.g., FFP) would contain anti-A antibodies. Since the red cells of type O recipients contain neither A nor B antigens, type O persons are "universal recipients" with regard to plasma. Type B plasma will contain anti-A antibodies. These antibodies will react with the A antigen on the AB recipient's red blood cells.

392. **The answer is C (2, 4).** Stoelting, *Anesthesia and Co-Existing Disease,* 3/e. pp 415–417.) The most common platelet disorder with massive blood transfusions is a dilutional thrombocytopenia, which can be corrected with platelet replacement. Inhibition of platelet cyclooxygenase by aspirin, which leads to thromboxane formation, occurs immediately after aspirin ingestion and affects the platelets exposed to aspirin for the duration of their lifetime. Once aspirin is stopped, newly formed platelets and transfused platelets will not be affected. Factor VIII deficiency, which occurs in von Willebrand's disease, produces impaired platelet aggregation. Platelets are damaged on transit through the oxygenator; the degree of damage parallels the duration of the cardiopulmonary bypass procedure. Platelet dysfunction quickly resolves after discontinuation of cardiopulmonary bypass.

393. **The answer is D (4).** (Stoelting, *Anesthesia and Co-Existing Disease,* 3/e. p 419.) The normal platelet life span is 9 to 11 days. ABO antigens probably are absorbed from plasma and are clinically insignificant; platelet-specific antigens and HLA antigens are more important. However, red cell "contamination" of platelet concentrates makes it wise not to give platelets from an Rh-positive donor to an Rh-negative female of childbearing age. Platelets are stored at 20 to 24°C. Because of higher storage temperatures, the risk of bacterial growth, and therefore infection, is higher.

394. The answer is C (2, 4). (Stoelting, *Anesthesia and Co-Existing Disease,* 3/e. pp 420–425.) Erythema and urticaria indicate an *allergic* reaction to infused blood. With a hemolytic reaction, it is important to stop the infusion of blood as soon as possible because morbidity (renal failure) is related to the volume infused. Unfortunately, in an anesthetized patient the only symptoms of a hemolytic reaction (back pain, fever, shivering, agitation) are unavailable. Unexplained hemorrhage and hemoglobinuria are later signs. Meperidine is helpful in treating shivering secondary to a febrile reaction.

395. The answer is D (4). (Stoelting, *Anesthesia and Co-Existing Disease,* 3/e. pp 420–425.) The transfusion should be stopped immediately if a hemolytic transfusion reaction is suspected. A patient with blood type A can receive packed red blood cells from an O donor but not fresh frozen plasma, since the plasma from a type O person has anti-A antibodies. Common intraoperative signs of a hemolytic transfusion reaction are hemoglobinuria, bleeding diathesis, and hypotension. Unfortunately, the use of donor-designated blood has not decreased the incidence of infection caused by blood transfusion. Most complications with transfusions are due to clerical error.

396. The answer is A (1, 2, 3). (Miller, 4/e. pp 1633–1635.) The most serious reactions involve intravascular hemolysis. Crystalloid should be infused to maintain urine output.

397. The answer is A (1, 2, 3). (Stoelting, *Anesthesia and Co-Existing Disease,* 3/e. pp 412–413.) Von Willebrand's disease is inherited in an autosomal dominant fashion. The deficient protein, termed *von Willebrand's factor (vWF),* participates in platelet activity and factor VIII function. Decreased plasma concentration of factor VIII, prolonged bleeding time, and poor platelet aggregation are manifestations. The treatment of bleeding secondary to von Willebrand's disease is with cryoprecipitate, which contains vWF. Factor VIII concentrates alone are not helpful.

398. The answer is C (2, 4). (Stoelting, *Anesthesia and Co-Existing Disease,* 3/e. pp 412–413.) Von Willebrand's disease is a defect in a protein that is important for optimal activity of factor VIII and platelets. Patients with this disease have low levels of factor VIII, elevated bleeding times, and dysfunctional platelet adhesiveness. Bleeding from mucosal surfaces (nosebleeds) and easy bruising are common. Treatment with factor VIII alone is inadequate. Desmopressin (a synthetic analogue of ADH known as *DDAVP*) induces the release of von Willebrand's factor and may be all that is necessary to improve platelet function and factor VIII function. If this treatment is inadequate, treatment with cryoprecipitate, which contains von Willebrand's factor, is indicated.

399. The answer is A (1, 2, 3). (Stoelting, *Anesthesia and Co-Existing Disease,* 3/e. p 396.) Hemoglobin A normally is composed of two alpha- and two beta-globin chains. Beta thalassemia is a relative or absolute deficiency of beta-globin chains. However, because they possess hemoglobin F, which is composed of two alpha- and two gamma-globin chains, newborns with beta thalassemia are not initially affected. Beta thalassemia major (Cooley's anemia) is a severe anemia that first manifests in infancy. Complications include hepatomegaly, splenomegaly, skeletal abnormalities, spinal cord compression, dysrhythmias, and congestive heart failure.

400. **The answer is A (1, 2, 3).** (Stoelting, *Anesthesia and Co-Existing Disease,* 3/e. pp 411–412.) The trait for hemophilia A is carried on the X chromosome. Hemophilia A results from decreased factor VIII activity. In addition to hemarthroses, hematuria, and deep tissue bleeding, a major cause of morbidity and mortality in patients with hemophilia A is central nervous system hemorrhage. Spontaneous hemorrhage is thought to occur when factor VIII levels reach 1 percent or less. The prothrombin time is normal in patients with hemophilia A. The partial thromboplastin time is a more useful screening test.

401. **The answer is B (1, 3).** (Stoelting, *Anesthesia and Co-Existing Disease,* 3/e. p 412.) Clinical features of hemophilia B are indistinguishable from those of hemophilia A. The combination of purpura, petechiae, and epistaxis is more characteristic of platelet dysfunction. Partial thromboplastin time is prolonged in hemophilia B. The treatment of choice is not FFP but specific factor IX concentrates.

402. **The answer is A (1, 2, 3).** (Stoelting, *Anesthesia and Co-Existing Disease,* 3/e. pp 401–403.) Prevention of acidosis and hypoxia is essential as sickling increases under these conditions. Hypovolemia may lead to circulatory stasis, as may hypothermia and the vasoconstriction that goes with it. Exchange transfusions are not done routinely. When they are done, hemoglobin A should be increased to 40 percent.

403. **The answer is A (1, 2, 3).** (Stoelting, *Anesthesia and Co-Existing Disease,* 3/e. pp 401–403.) Sickling of cells is favored by conditions of decreased oxygen tension and pH. Hence, there is a greater propensity for sickling in veins as opposed to arteries and for infarction in the renal medulla, an area of low oxygen tension.

404. **The answer is C (2, 4).** (Stoelting, *Anesthesia and Co-Existing Disease,* 3/e. pp 401–403.) In sickle cell trait, sickling occurs under extreme hypoxic conditions, i.e., at a Pa_{O_2} in the range of 20 to 30 mmHg. In sickle cell disease, by contrast, sickling can occur as Pa_{O_2} drops below 40 mmHg. Therefore, sickling occurs at a normal venous Pa_{O_2}. Good anesthetic care consists of careful ventilatory management to avoid acidosis and careful attention to volume status as well as avoidance of hypothermia. The listed problems with use of a tourniquet are possible and should be given consideration, but tourniquets have been used successfully in patients with sickle cell disease and are not absolutely contraindicated. Chronic pulmonary infarcts lead to poor ventilation-perfusion mismatching and abnormalities of diffusing capacity.

405. **The answer is C (2, 4).** (Stoelting, *Anesthesia and Co-Existing Disease,* 3/e. p 403.) In methemoglobin iron exists in the ferric rather than ferrous form. The ferric form is not able to bind oxygen. Methemoglobin shifts the oxyhemoglobin dissociation curve to the left and decreases the amount of oxygen unloaded to tissues. Cyanosis occurs usually with 5 g/dL of deoxygenated hemoglobin. It occurs with 1.5 g/dL of methemoglobin. Nitrate-containing substances may lead to an increase in methemoglobin, especially in persons missing the enzyme methemoglobin reductase.

EYES

Directions: Each question below contains four suggested responses of which **one or more** is correct. Select

(A)	if	**1, 2, and 3**	are correct
(B)	if	**1 and 3**	are correct
(C)	if	**2 and 4**	are correct
(D)	if	**4**	is correct
(E)	if	**1, 2, 3, and 4**	are correct

406. Echothiophate iodide eye drops act systematically to

(1) decrease minimum alveolar concentration (MAC)
(2) antagonize opioids
(3) act as a beta-adrenergic receptor blocking drug
(4) reduce pseudocholinesterase activity

407. Decreases in intraocular pressure are associated with

(1) hypothermia
(2) the administration of opioids
(3) the administration of etomidate
(4) hypoventilation

408. The oculocardiac reflex may be elicited by

(1) pressure on the globe
(2) traction on extraocular muscles
(3) development of an orbital hematoma
(4) occurrence of tachycardia and hypertension on induction

409. True statements with regard to oculocardiac reflex include

(1) it can be both elicited and attenuated by performance of retrobulbar block

(2) its afferent limb is the trigeminal nerve, and its efferent limb is the vagal nerve

(3) its occurrence is higher in the pediatric patient

(4) pretreatment with an anticholinergic agent is the most effective treatment

410. Injection of a small bubble of gas into the vitreal cavity during retinal surgery will

(1) repair the optic nerve

(2) decrease the specific gravity of vitreous content

(3) keep the eye immobile postoperatively

(4) hold the repaired retina in place

411. With respect to intraocular injection of sulfur hexafluoride (SF_6), true statements include

(1) it is used in retinal reattachment surgery

(2) nitrous oxide should be discontinued for at least 15 min before injection of SF_6 to prevent expansion of the gas bubble

(3) SF has a lower blood-gas partition coefficient than do nitrogen and nitrous oxide

(4) if reoperation is required, nitrous oxide can be safety used 48 h after intravitreous injection of SF_6

412. In anesthetic management for strabismus surgery, one should remember that

(1) an increased susceptibility to malignant hyperthermia exists

(2) oculocardiac reflex occurs during surgery

(3) the existence of oculogastric reflex predisposes to the development of postoperative vomiting

(4) administration of droperidol before manipulation of the eye muscles has been shown to prevent postoperative vomiting completely

413. True statements about drugs and their effects on the eyes include

(1) pilocarpine, used in the treatment of glaucoma, produces dilated pupils

(2) timolol, when applied topically to the eyes, may produce signs of cardiac or pulmonary beta blockade

(3) plasma cholinesterase activity returns to normal 4 to 7 days after stopping echothiophate eyedrops

(4) normal intraocular pressure is 10 to 20 mmHg

414. Major considerations for emergency anesthesia in a patient with an open-globe eye injury include

(1) prevention of aspiration

(2) prevention of an increase in intraocular pressure during induction and maintenance

(3) blocking the cardiovascular response to intubation

(4) prevention of sepsis postoperatively

EYES

406. **The answer is D (4).** (Miller, 4/e. p 2183.) Echothiophate iodide eye drops, when absorbed systemically, reduce the activity of pseudocholinesterase. Echothiophate is a long-acting anticholinesterase that irreversibly binds to pseudocholinesterase and renders it totally inactive. This action can last for 4 to 6 weeks after discontinuation of echothiophate and can prolong the effects of succinylcholine and ester local anesthetics.

407. **The answer is A (1, 2, 3).** (Miller, 4/e. pp 2177–2179.) Among the listed factors, only hypoventilation has been shown to increase intraocular pressure.

408. **The answer is A (1, 2, 3).** (Miller, 4/e. p 2182.) The oculocardiac reflex is a trigeminal-vagal reflex. It most commonly causes bradycardia and nodal rhythms. Asystole, ectopy, and ventricular fibrillation also may occur. In addition to the listed causes, ocular trauma and ocular pain can elicit this reflex. Tachycardia and hypertension do not.

409. **The answer is A (1, 2, 3).** (Barash, 3/e. p 916.) Pretreatment with an anticholinergic agent has not been found to be effective in the treatment of oculocardiac reflex. Treatment with atropine after the reflex has occurred usually will resolve the problem quickly.

410. **The answer is D (4).** (Miller, 4/e. p 2179.) Injection of a gas bubble into the vitreous cavity aids retinal repair. The gases most commonly used are sulfur hexafluoride (SF_6) and carbon octofluoride (C_3F_8). These gases are inert, insoluble in water, and poorly diffusible.

411. **The answer is A (1, 2, 3).** (Miller, 4/e. p 2179.) Nitrous oxide may rapidly enter these gas bubbles and expand volume and increase ocular pressure. These changes in bubble size and intraocular pressure can jeopardize a retinal repair. It is recommended to discontinue use of N_2O 20 min before gas injection or not to use N_2O at all. If reoperation is required, it is recommended that nitrous oxide not be used until 10 days after intravitreous injection of SF_6 and 5 days after intravitreous injection of air.

412. **The answer is A (1, 2, 3).** (Miller, 4/e. pp 2181–2182.) Although administration of droperidol before manipulation of the eye muscles has been shown to decrease the incidence of postoperative vomiting, it does not prevent its occurrence completely.

413. **The answer is C (2, 4).** (Miller, 4/e. p 2183.) Parasympathomimetics, used in the treatment of glaucoma, include pilocarpine and echothiophate. These drugs produce miosis. Normal activity does not return until about 4 weeks after stopping echothiophate. Topical application of timolol can produce bradycardia, hypotension, and bronchospasm by systemic absorption. An intraocular pressure ≥ 25 mmHg is pathologic.

414. **The answer is A (1, 2, 3).** (Miller, 4/e. pp 2179–2180.) The use of H_2 blockers, metoclopramide, a nonparticulate antacid, and the Sellick maneuver may help limit or prevent passive regurgitation. Increases in intraocular pressure (IOP) may cause extrusion of vitreous and thus worsen the injury. Coughing or bucking on the tube at any point during the surgery and emesis postoperatively may cause an increase in IOP. Blocking the cardiovascular response to intubation is especially important in patients with coronary disease and may be especially challenging when one is trying to induce anesthesia quickly and deeply to avoid aspiration and increases in IOP.

GERIATRICS

Directions: Each question below contains four suggested responses of which **one or more** is correct. Select

(A)	if	**1, 2, and 3**	are correct
(B)	if	**1 and 3**	are correct
(C)	if	**2 and 4**	are correct
(D)	if	**4**	is correct
(E)	if	**1, 2, 3, and 4**	are correct

415. Considerations in elderly patients include that

(1) body fat decreases, as does the half-life of fat-soluble drugs

(2) impaired hypothalamic function, which mediates heat control, is the primary reason the elderly become hypothermic more easily than do the young

(3) right bundle branch blocks are common in healthy, asymptomatic elderly patients and in most cases should be considered a normal finding

(4) they have a widened pulse pressure

416. Important pharmacologic considerations in the elderly include that

(1) the dose of thiopental in elderly patients should be decreased primarily because of altered pharmacokinetics

(2) the elimination half-life of diazepam in hours approximates the patient's age in years

(3) the dose of atracurium need not be adjusted for age

(4) the MAC for isoflurane in a 40-year-old is 1.15 and in an 80-year-old is 0.97

417. Changes in cardiac output in the elderly are correctly characterized by which of the following statements?

 (1) Cardiac output declines more with age in women than in men
 (2) Increases in cardiac output that occur with stress decline with aging
 (3) Coronary blood flow needs are decreased in the elderly for a given cardiac output
 (4) Persons who maintain physical aerobic fitness may have unchanged cardiac output from the third to the sixth decade

418. True statements about the hepatobiliary system in the geriatric age group include

 (1) hepatic blood flow decreases as a result of decreased cardiac output
 (2) a decrease in activity of hepatic microsomal enzymes occurs
 (3) production of albumin is decreased
 (4) hepatic vein blood flow decreases

419. Which of the following changes in renal function will occur in the geriatric population?

 (1) An increase in renal cortical blood flow versus renal medullary blood flow occurs
 (2) Decreased muscle mass in the elderly leads to decreased creatinine levels
 (3) There are no changes in urine concentrating ability
 (4) Decreased renal blood flow occurs because of decreased cardiac output and a decrease in size of the renal vascular bed

420. Changes in cardiac physiology that occur in the elderly include

 (1) a decrease in beta receptor responsiveness but no change in receptor density
 (2) increased responsiveness of the geriatric heart to indirect-acting beta mimetics such as ephedrine
 (3) degenerative changes of the SA node, AV node, and cardiac conduction system
 (4) higher resting heart rates

421. Ventilatory function is impaired in the elderly for which of the following reasons?

 (1) Decreased intercostal and diaphragmatic muscle mass and function
 (2) Loss of alveolar spaces and septa, which resembles emphysematous changes
 (3) Decreased pulmonary parenchymal and chest wall elasticity
 (4) Diminished hypoxic drive

422. Endocrinologic changes that occur in the elderly include

 (1) a greater incidence of primary hyperparathyroidism
 (2) increased incidence of diabetes mellitus
 (3) increased incidence of Graves' disease
 (4) increased incidence of hypothyroidism

423. Major anatomic changes seen in the cardiovascular system in the elderly include

(1) an increase in left ventricular wall thickness
(2) myocardial fibrosis
(3) valvular fibrocalcifications
(4) loss of elasticity of the peripheral circulation

424. Airway changes that occur in the elderly include

(1) endentulousness, which causes difficulties with mask ventilation
(2) cervical and temperomandibular joint osteoarthritis
(3) vertebrobasilar and carotid artery insufficiency, which can become symptomatic upon rotation of the head
(4) weakening of the posterior wall of the trachea, which leads to a greater potential for perforation

425. True statements concerning the elderly include

(1) there is a direct correlation between biologic age and chronologic age
(2) the five most frequently performed surgical procedures are cataract extraction, transurethral prostatectomy, herniorrhaphy, cholecystectomy, and reduction of a hip fracture
(3) geriatric patients are arbitrarily defined as those older than 75 years of age
(4) generalized osteoporosis may be an important factor in the increased incidence of hip fractures in the elderly

426. Changes in the central nervous system (CNS) that occur in the geriatric population include

(1) a progressive decline in CNS function with a loss of cerebral cortex neurons
(2) decreased cerebral metabolic rate and decreased cerebral blood flow
(3) a decrease in the synthesis of neurotransmitters and receptor sites for them
(4) a need for increased doses of local anesthetics when epidural anesthesia is performed

GERIATRICS

ANSWERS

415. **The answer is D (4).** (Stoelting, *Anesthesia and Co-Existing Disease,* 3/e. pp 631–633.) Body fat increases (in women more than in men) and fat-soluble drugs have a longer elimination half-life in the elderly. Hypothalamic dysfunction may be one factor that contributes to a greater degree of heat loss in elderly patients, but the primary reason for a propensity to hypothermia is impaired cutaneous vasoconstriction and reduced heat production (basal metabolic rate declines from 42 kcal/h in a 20-year-old to 32 kcal/h in an 80-year-old person). Healthy, asymptomatic elderly patients have a high incidence of supraventricular and ventricular ectopic beats. A right bundle branch block is not a normal finding and should prompt a search for organic heart disease. Systolic blood pressure increases in the elderly as the aorta and large arteries lose distensibility. Diastolic pressure normally does not change much with age.

416. **The answer is E (all).** (Miller, 4/e. pp 2143–2146.) The initial volume of distribution for thiopental is decreased, which causes higher serum concentrations in older compared with younger patients. Elderly and younger patients respond to similar serum concentrations of thiopental. The clearance of diazepam is reduced in the elderly, which accounts for its longer duration of action. Cognitive impairment can continue for a very long time after administration of this drug in the elderly. Unlike all other nondepolarizing muscle relaxants, atracurium is independent of age-related changes. Decreases in MAC occur with age for isoflurane and the other potent inhalational agents.

417. **The answer is C (2, 4).** (Miller, 4/e. pp 2150–2151.) Cardiac output does not necessarily decline with aging. Persons who maintain aerobic fitness may have unchanged cardiac output well into the seventh decade, at which point cardiac output will fall off. In the elderly there is a loss of an increase in cardiac output in response to stress, but this is attenuated somewhat in the elderly who are fit.

418. **The answer is E (all).** (Miller, 4/e. pp 2145–2146.) The reduction in hepatic blood flow is commensurate with the decrease in cardiac output that occurs in the elderly. Hepatic microsomal enzyme activity also decreases in the aged. Drug clearance and metabolism are reduced in the elderly, but the cause of this is probably the decrease in cardiac output rather than diminished enzyme activity. Hepatic vein blood flow and albumin levels are diminished in the elderly.

419. **The answer is C (2, 4).** (Miller, 4/e. pp 2146–2147.) Renal blood flow decreases in the elderly because of a decrease in cardiac output and a decrease in the size of the renal vasculature, particularly the cortex. This leads to reduced renal cortical blood flow and decreased glomerular filtration rate (GFR), concentrating ability, and creatinine clearance. With the decrease in creatinine clearance, there is also a decrease in muscle mass and production of creatinine. This explains why serum creatinine levels do not decrease in the elderly. Any increase in creatinine in the elderly signifies a large decrease in an already diminished GFR.

420. **The answer is B (1, 3).** (Miller, 4/e. pp 2150–2151.) There is no change in beta receptor density in the elderly; however, function is diminished, which affects inotropicity and chronotropicity. Also, as a result of diminished function, there is diminished responsiveness to both direct and indirect beta sympathomimetic drugs. There are degenerative fibrotic changes throughout the conduction system, which can lead to heart blocks. Resting heart rate is decreased.

421. **The answer is E (all).** (Miller, 4/e. 2151–2152.) Hypoxic and carbon dioxide drive is not lost in the elderly, but it may be diminished. Therefore, the elderly are at great risk for hypoxia and hypercarbia from anesthetic drugs that cause respiratory depression. Another factor adding to potential pulmonary failure in the elderly is complex mechanical changes that involve the chest wall, diaphragm, and pulmonary parenchyma.

422. **The answer is C (2, 4).** (Stoelting, *Anesthesia and Co-Existing Disease,* 3/e. pp 633–636.) Primary hyperparathyroidism and Graves' disease do not have an increased incidence in the elderly. Adult-onset diabetes occurs with greater frequency in the sixth and seventh decades. Circulating insulin levels are normal. It is believed that the cause of diabetes in this age group may be insulin receptor dysfunction. Thirteen percent of the elderly population have hypothyroidism; the vast majority are asymptomatic. The only abnormal measure of thyroid function may be an elevated level of thyroid stimulating hormone. The most common cause of hypothyroidism is Hashimoto's thyroiditis.

423. **The answer is E (all).** (Miller, 4/e. pp 2150–2151.) All the listed changes are normal parts of the aging process. Atherosclerosis superimposed on these changes only exacerbates the decrease in cardiovascular function, particularly a decrease in cardiac output.

424. The answer is E (all). (Stoelting, *Anesthesia and Co-Existing Disease,* 3/e. p. 634.) Airway evaluation in the elderly is extremely important. Leaving dentures in place may make mask ventilation easier. Head positioning and mask airway intubation conditions are made more difficult because of underlying osteoarthritis of both the cervical spine and the temperomandibular joints. These patients may have variable degrees of osteoporosis of the cervical spine and are at increased risk for fractures with forceful movement of the head. Because of diffuse atherosclerosis, vertebrobasilar and carotid artery stenosis can occur, which may be symptomatic only with extreme ranges of motion of the head. This may manifest as transient ischemic attacks or even strokes from atherosclerotic emboli.

425. The answer is C (2, 4). (Stoelting, *Anesthesia and Co-Existing Disease,* 2/e. pp 633–637.) There is no definite correlation between biologic age and chronologic age. In patients who maintain aerobic fitness, there may be no changes in cardiac output until well into the seventh decade. Physical fitness will even decrease osteoporosis and may cause a decrease in the incidence of hip fractures. Patients who do not maintain aerobic fitness may show signs of osteoporosis and decreases in cardiac output that make them biologically older than those who do. Geriatric patients are arbitrarily defined as those over 65 years of age.

426. The answer is A (1, 2, 3). (Miller, 4/e. pp 2147–2148.) There is a generalized decline in the CNS with aging. MAC decreases as a result. Local anesthetic requirements decrease as well as for all nerve blocks.

PEDIATRICS

DIRECTIONS: Each question below contains four or five suggested responses. Select the **one best** response to each question.

427. All the following statements concerning the fetal hematologic system are true EXCEPT

  (A) physiologic anemia occurs at 1 month of age

  (B) fetal hemoglobin has P-50 of 19 mmHg compared with 26 mmHg for adult hemoglobin

  (C) fetal hemoglobin has a greater affinity for O_2, and this manifests as decreased O_2 delivery to the periphery compared with adult hemoglobin

  (D) the decreased P-50 of fetal hemoglobin causes a shift to the left of the oxygen dissociation curve

  (E) decreased release of oxygen by fetal hemoglobin is offset by increased oxygen delivery provided by elevated hemoglobin concentrations in neonates

428. The glomerular filtration rate reaches that of the adult by age

  (A) 1 month

  (B) 6 months

  (C) 1 year

  (D) 18 months

  (E) 2 years

429. The following statements about thermoregulation in the neonate are all true EXCEPT

  (A) neonates have a larger body surface area compared with body weight than do adults

  (B) neonates have mature central thermoregulatory control

  (C) neonates have a specialized ability to produce heat

  (D) neonates have a very thin layer of subcutaneous fat

  (E) neonates cannot shiver to produce heat

430. Normal fetal circulation is characterized by all the following EXCEPT

(A) high pulmonary vascular resistance
(B) low systemic vascular resistance
(C) right-to-left shunting of blood through the foramen ovale
(D) right-to-left shunting of blood through a ventricular septal defect (VSD) that closes functionally soon after delivery
(E) right-to-left shunting of blood via the ductus arteriosus

431. Onset of spontaneous ventilation at birth causes all the following EXCEPT

(A) a decrease in pulmonary vascular resistance
(B) an increase in systemic vascular resistance
(C) an increase in left atrial pressure with a functional closure of the foramen ovale
(D) anatomic closure of the foramen ovale 1 month after birth
(E) functional closure of the ductus arteriosus 10 to 15 h after birth

432. With regard to the fetal circulation,

(A) the right ventricle ejects one-third of the ventricular output
(B) it is arranged in series
(C) placental blood is well oxygenated
(D) 50 percent of the blood entering the pulmonary artery is shunted to the aorta

433. Cardiovascular responses of neonates differ from those of adults in all the following ways EXCEPT

(A) neonates have greater myocardial collateral blood flow
(B) neonates have less cardiac compliance
(C) reductions in heart rate significantly decrease neonatal cardiac output compared with that in adults
(D) an immature sympathetic nervous system innervates the fetal myocardium
(E) neonates have less vasoconstriction in response to hemorrhage

434. Before anesthesia neonates should

(A) fast for 2 h
(B) fast for 4 h
(C) fast for 6 h
(D) fast for 8 h
(E) not fast because gastric emptying is slow and liver glycogen stores are low

435. A 10-kg child has been NPO for 4 h. During the first hour of surgery, the amount of intravenous fluid the child should receive is

(A) 40 mL
(B) 80 mL
(C) 100 mL
(D) 120 mL
(E) 160 mL

436. Which of the following statements pertaining to control of ventilation in neonates is true?

(A) Hypoxia leads to sustained hyperventilation

(B) Hypercarbia leads to sustained hyperventilation

(C) The ventilatory response to hypercarbia in newborns is mature at birth

(D) With both hypoxia and hypercarbia, newborns respond initially by hyperventilating but then start to hypoventilate

(E) None of the above

437. You are the anesthesiologist attending the vaginal delivery of a full-term newborn. Arterial blood gas sampled immediately at delivery shows the following: pH = 7.25, P_{CO_2} = 50, P_{O_2} = 50. Which course of action is indicated?

(A) Establishment of venous access, administration of 1 meq/kg $NaHCO_3$

(B) Positive pressure ventilation with 100% O_2 by mask

(C) Immediate orotracheal intubation

(D) Gentle suction and stimulation; keep baby warm; no resuscitation needed

Directions: Each question below contains four suggested responses of which **one or more** is correct. Select

(A)	if	**1, 2, and 3**	are correct
(B)	if	**1 and 3**	are correct
(C)	if	**2 and 4**	are correct
(D)	if	**4**	is correct
(E)	if	**1, 2, 3, and 4**	are correct

438. True statements concerning fluid and electrolyte management in pediatric patients include which of the following?

(1) Because of the greater hypoxic damage associated with high blood glucose levels and the infrequent occurrence of hypoglycemia in newborns, administration of a dextrose-containing solution is not recommended

(2) During the first days of life, term newborns need a larger volume of maintenance fluid per kilogram of body weight than do older children

(3) Replacement fluid for deficit and third-space loss should be hypotonic given the inability of young infants to handle an excess sodium load

(4) To minimize dehydration, restriction of fluids in a neonate should be less than 2 to 4 h

439. The delivery of a hypotonic newborn after cesarean section may have resulted from administration to the mother of

(1) 30 min 70% nitrous oxide
(2) 5 mg/kg thiopental
(3) 1% isoflurane
(4) 1.5 mg/kg ketamine

440. Normal values for a full-term 1-day-old neonate include

(1) a hemoglobin of 16 to 18
(2) an estimated blood volume of 80 to 85 mL/kg
(3) a distance between lips and midtrachea of 10 cm
(4) a systolic blood pressure of 60 mmHg

441. True statements about a full-term neonate include

(1) a normal systolic blood pressure is 60 to 65 torr
(2) the ratio of body surface area to volume is increased, and so heat loss to the environment is increased
(3) a 3.0 should be the first size of endotracheal tube attempted
(4) in a neonate vital capacity and functional residual capacity are increased compared with an adult

442. Proper care of a neonate at birth includes knowledge of which of the following facts?

(1) Every neonate born with meconium-stained amniotic fluid should be intubated and suctioned through an endotracheal tube

(2) The ductus arteriosus of a term neonate is not fully anatomically closed until age 10 to 14 days

(3) Apgar scores assess five features of the newborn: respirations, heart rate, color, muscle tone, and reflex irritability

(4) A normal respiratory rate within moments of birth is 25 to 30 breaths per minute

443. True statements concerning congenital diaphragmatic hernia (CDH) include

(1) the degree of hypoplastic lung tissue or abnormal pulmonary vascular development is an important indicator for prognosis

(2) awake intubation is the best choice for securing the airway

(3) positive pressure ventilation by mask should be avoided

(4) the development of pneumothorax in the lung contralateral to the hernia is a frequent complication

444. Tracheoesophageal fistula may be associated with

(1) vertebral anomalies

(2) anal anomalies

(3) renal anomalies

(4) congenital heart disease

445. Regarding congenital diaphragmatic hernias,

(1) the arterial hypoxemia usually seen in these neonates is due to severe ventilation-perfusion mismatch in the abnormal lung

(2) the presenting symptoms include respiratory distress, cyanosis, and a scaphoid abdomen

(3) initial management of a newborn in severe respiratory distress with a suspected diagnosis of diaphragmatic hernia consists of gentle positive pressure ventilation via face mask with 100% oxygen

(4) airway pressure during mechanical ventilation should not exceed 30 cmH_2O because of the risk of pneumothorax on the side opposite to that of the hernia

446. The ductus arteriosus will close in term animals in response to

(1) oxygen

(2) parasympathetic stimulation

(3) acetylcholine

(4) prostaglandins

447. True statements regarding hypercyanotic attacks in patients with tetralogy of Fallot ("tet spells") include

  (1) they are often associated with agitation

  (2) squatting is thought to increase systemic vascular resistance and thereby improve blood flow into the systemic circulation

  (3) 3 to 5 μg/kg of phenylephrine given as a bolus is one of the recommended treatments

  (4) positive end-expiratory pressure and slight underventilation of the lungs during mechanical ventilation would be expected to improve oxygenation during an intraoperative onset

448. True statements with regard to the induction of anesthesia in an infant with tetralogy of Fallot include which of the following?

  (1) Inhalational induction with halothane and nitrous oxide would be expected to be more rapid because of the presence of a right-to-left shunt

  (2) Less than 50 μg/kg of fentanyl should be used because of possible profound cardiovascular effects in an infant

  (3) Halothane is the preferred anesthetic agent because it is much less cardiodepressant in infants than in adults

  (4) The maintenance of airway patency and adequate ventilation is important in minimizing the increase in pulmonary vascular resistance, irrespective of the induction technique

SUMMARY OF DIRECTIONS

A	B	C	D	E
1,2,3 only	1,3 only	2,4 only	4 only	All are correct

449. True statements about fetal monitoring during labor include

(1) late decelerations that occur at the end of uterine contractions are thought to indicate compromised oxygen supply to the fetus
(2) variable decelerations are thought to represent compression of the fetal head
(3) early decelerations are not associated with compromised fetuses
(4) if a fetal scalp sample shows a P_{O_2} of 25 mmHg, this is an indication for emergency cesarean section

450. In comparison with the airway anatomy of an adult, a pediatric patient has

(1) a smaller tongue relative to total body size
(2) a larger mouth relative to total body size
(3) a larynx that is widest at the cricoid cartilage
(4) a larynx more anteriorly displaced

451. Severe hypovolemia in a neonate is indicated by

(1) a warm entire extremity
(2) absent posterior tibial pulse
(3) capillary refill in less than 2 s
(4) mottled appearing skin

452. True statements concerning pulmonary physiology in newborns include

(1) carbon dioxide production is less in a newborn than in an adult
(2) oxygen consumption in newborns is double that of adults, 6 mL/kg/min versus 3 mL/kg/min
(3) minute ventilation based on milliliters per kilogram per minute is the same in newborns and adults
(4) tidal volumes based on milliliters per kilogram are the same, but the respiratory rate is double in a newborn compared with an adult

453. Pediatric cardiopulmonary bypass (CPB) differs from adult CPB in that in the former

(1) deeper hypothermia is used
(2) lower perfusion pressures are used
(3) hemodilution is greater
(4) pump flow rates vary more widely

454. True statements regarding sodium bicarbonate include that it

(1) should be given in neonatal resuscitation
(2) may result in intraventricular hemorrhage in premature infants
(3) is useful in the treatment of respiratory acidosis
(4) may lead to hypotension when given to neonates

455. Features of pyloric stenosis include

(1) loss of gastric HCl
(2) metabolic alkalosis
(3) dehydration
(4) respiratory alkalosis

456. In a 4-year-old patient who is returning from the recovery room to the operating room for control of surgical bleeding after tonsillectomy, important concerns include that

    (1)   the patient should be considered to have a full stomach

    (2)   an inhalational induction is contraindicated

    (3)   the patient may be hypovolemic

    (4)   succinylcholine is contraindicated in this age group because of the risk of masseter spasm and malignant hyperthermia

457. Patients with pyloric stenosis

    (1)   constitute a surgical emergency

    (2)   present frequently between 3 and 6 weeks of age

    (3)   manifest a hyperchloremic, hyperkalemic, metabolic alkalosis

    (4)   are dehydrated

458. True statements regarding epiglottitis include which of the following?

    (1)   It occurs most commonly in children age 3 months to 3 years

    (2)   The disease is not seen in neonates or the elderly

    (3)   Observation of a child with suspected epiglottitis in a quiet area and administration of racemic epinephrine constitute adequate management provided that respiratory distress is absent on initial presentation

    (4)   The recent introduction of the *Haemophilus influenzae* vaccine may make classic cases of epiglottitis much less common

459. In an infant,

    (1)   the narrowest part of the trachea is at the cricoid

    (2)   alveoli increase in size and number until 1 year of age and increase only in size afterward

    (3)   dead space ventilation is similar to that in an adult

    (4)   closing capacity is less than functional residual capacity (FRC)

460. Down's syndrome is associated with

    (1)   a high incidence of congenital heart defects

    (2)   upper and lower airway abnormalities

    (3)   cervical neck instability

    (4)   sensitivity to atropine

461. In a neonate

    (1)   the percentage of total body water is greater than in an adult

    (2)   the volume of distribution of water-soluble drugs is greater than in an adult

    (3)   renal function is diminished, impairing the ability to handle free water and solutes

    (4)   drugs redistributed to the fat will have a longer clinical effect

462. The use of regional anesthesia in premature infants less than 60 weeks of postconceptual age has been advocated to reduce

    (1)   retinopathy of prematurity

    (2)   intracranial hemorrhage

    (3)   stress reaction to surgery

    (4)   postoperative apnea

PEDIATRICS

ANSWERS

427. The answer is A. (Stoelting, *Anesthesia and Co-Existing Disease,* 3/e. p 583.) There are differences between fetal hemoglobin and adult hemoglobin that influence O_2 transport and delivery. Fetal hemoglobin has a greater affinity for oxygen, which results in a lower P-50 (19 mmHg) and causes a shift to the left of the O_2 dissociation curve. For these reasons, there is decreased release of O_2 to the periphery. However, there is a greater amount of fetal hemoglobin, and this offsets the increased affinity by increasing delivery of O_2. Physiologic anemia occurs at about 2 to 3 months of age, when production of adult hemoglobin begin in earnest.

428. The answer is C. (Miller, 4/e. pp 2469–2470.) By age 1 year glomerular filtration reaches the adult rate.

429. The answer is B. (Stoelting, *Anesthesia and Co-Existing Disease,* 3/e. pp 583–584.) Neonates are particularly prone to hypothermia in the operating room as their central thermoregulatory controls are immature. They have a large ratio of body surface area to body weight and lose heat more quickly than adults do. Neonates also have less insulating subcutaneous fat than do adults. Infants do not shiver to produce heat. Heat is generated from the metabolism of the brown fat they possess. Methods to prevent heat loss in neonates include increasing the operating room temperature, warming fluids, heating and humidifying gases, covering exposed body surfaces, and using radiant-heat tables in the operating room.

430. The answer is D. (Stoelting, *Anesthesia and Co-Existing Disease,* 3/e. pp 37–38, 581–582.) A ventricular septal defect (VSD) is not a normal component of the fetal circulation pattern. VSDs constitute approximately 28 percent of congenital cardiac anomalies, and they are more common in premature infants. Twenty-eight percent of VSDs are small and will close spontaneously. The symptoms of a large VSD include tachypnea, tachycardia, failure to thrive, recurrent pulmonary infections, and ultimately congestive heart failure. If medical management is unsuccessful, surgical treatment, which depends on the type of VSD, is considered.

431. **The answer is D.** (Stoelting, *Anesthesia and Co-Existing Disease,* 3/e. p 581.) With the onset of spontaneous ventilation at birth, several events occur to convert fetal circulation to adult circulation. Pulmonary vascular resistance decreases because of increased FI_{O_2} and exhalation of lung water. Systemic vascular resistance increases after separation from the low vascular resistance of the placenta. As a result, there is an increase in pulmonary blood flow with a functional end to right-to-left shunting through both the ductus arteriosus and the foramen ovale. The higher left atrial pressures and resistances also diminish right-to-left shunting and aid in the increase in pulmonary blood flow. Functional closure of the ductus arteriosus occurs 10 to 15 h after birth; anatomic closure occurs in 4 to 6 weeks. The foramen ovale closes anatomically between 3 months and 1 year, although 20 to 30 percent of patients have probe-patent foramen ovales.

432. **The answer is C.** (Miller, 4/e. p 2078.) The right ventricle ejects two-thirds of the combined ventricular output. The *adult* circulation is arranged in series; the fetal circulation is in parallel. Blood returning from the placenta is well oxygenated. Approximately 95 percent of blood entering the pulmonary artery is shunted through the ductus arteriosus to the aorta.

433. **The answer is A.** (Stoelting, *Anesthesia and Co-Existing Disease,* 2/e. p 581. Miller, 4/e. pp 1812–1814, 2098–2099.) Neonates do not have greater collateral myocardial blood flow than adults. The adult heart has 60 percent contractile elements as opposed to 30 percent in the neonate. This means that for a given volume, less tension or pressure is generated in a neonate heart, which makes it less compliant. Neonates are dependent on maintenance of heart rate for stable cardiac output. The sympathetic nervous system of a neonate is immature and produces less vasoconstriction in response to hemorrhage.

434. **The answer is A.** (Firestone, 3/e. pp 390–391.) Before anesthesia neonates should have nothing by mouth for 2 h. The recommended fast is 4 h at 1 to 6 months, 6 h at 6 to 36 months, and 8 h at more than 36 months.

435. **The answer is D.** (Miller, 4/e. p 2112.) The child's hourly maintenance is 4 mL/kg, which at 10 kg is 40 mL. The 4-h deficit is thus 160 mL. During the first hour of surgery, the child should receive 50 percent of the deficit (80 mL) plus the hourly maintenance (40 mL) for a total of 120 mL.

436. **The answer is D.** (Stoelting, *Anesthesia and Co-Existing Disease,* 3/e. pp 579–580.) Control of ventilation in premature infants and neonates is immature. When neonates are subjected to hypoxia or hypercarbia, for 1 to 2 min, there is hyperventilation. After this time, the neonate will hypoventilate and may even become apneic. High levels of carbon dioxide may be a respiratory depressant in neonates. Respiratory depressants will act synergistically with the immature response to ventilation. It must also be remembered that oxygen consumption and carbon dioxide production in a neonate are double those in an adult.

437. **The answer is D.** (Barash, 3/e. p 1094.) The blood gas values are normal for a full-term newborn immediately after birth. No resuscitation is indicated.

438. **The answer is D (4).** (Miller, 4/e. pp 2108–2109, 2112–2113.) The greater hypoxic damage associated with high blood glucose levels has been shown only in animal studies. Hypoglycemia in newborns is a real concern. Therefore, administration of a dextrose-containing solution is recommended, but blood glucose levels should be monitored to prevent hyperglycemia. Term newborns do have a large ratio of body surface area to weight and a higher metabolic demand. Their maintenance fluid requirement, however, is usually lower during the first days of life because of their inability to excrete excess water. Replacement fluid for deficit and third-space loss should be an isotonic solution because of the inability of young infants to handle and eliminate excess free water load; they are better able to handle an excess sodium load.

439. **The answer is A (1, 2, 3).** (Miller, 4/e. pp 2044, 2059–2061.) Long exposure to nitrous oxide, inhalational agents, and thiopental more than 4 mg/kg can all depress a newborn. In contrast, more than 1 mg/kg of ketamine produces hypertonia in a newborn.

440. **The answer is E (all).** (Stoelting, *Anesthesia and Co-Existing Disease,* 3/e. pp 580–583.) All these answers are true. Neonatal hemoglobin is primarily fetal hemoglobin, which gradually disappears over the first 3 months of life.

441. **The answer is A (1, 2, 3).** (Stoelting, *Anesthesia and Co-Existing Disease,* 3/e. pp 579–582.) The ratio of body surface area to volume is increased, which accounts for the increased heat loss from a neonate. A 3.0 should be the first size of endotracheal tube attempted in a term neonate; the average distance from lips to midtrachea is 10 cm. Respiratory rate and carbon dioxide production are increased, but functional residual capacity and vital capacity are smaller compared with an adult.

442. **The answer is A (1, 2, 3).** (Miller, 4/e. pp 2079–2081, 2086.) Meconium may move to alveoli and may cause respiratory difficulties if it is not suctioned. Exposure of the neonate during this time to hypoxia, acidosis, or cold can revert the circulation to the fetal form with shunting of blood across the ductus arteriosus and resultant hypoxemia. A normal respiratory rate is 30 to 60 breaths per minute. Slow respiratory rates can indicate acidosis, asphyxia, maternal drug effect, or severe infection.

443. **The answer is E (all).** (Barash, 3/e. pp 1103–1104.) Mortality is still quite high with this disease. Intrauterine diagnosis can help one plan treatment prophylactically.

444. **The answer is E (all).** (Miller, 4/e. pp 2118–2119.) Tracheoesophageal fistula may be associated with anomalies in all the systems. This group of anomalies is referred to as the *VATER syndrome: V,* vertebral; *A,* anal; *TE,* tracheoesophageal fistula; *R,* renal anomalies.

445. **The answer is C (2, 4).** (Barash, 3/e. pp 1103–1104. Stoelting, *Anesthesia and Co-Existing Disease,* 3/e. pp 591–593.) The arterial hypoxemia in these patients is most often due to persistent fetal circulation across a patent ductus arteriosus, which persists because of increased pulmonary vascular resistance, acidosis, hypoxemia, and hypercapnia. Pulmonary hypoplasia is another cause of hypoxemia. The abdomen is usually scaphoid, since abdominal contents have shifted into the thorax. Cyanosis and respiratory distress are commonly seen. Bowel sounds sometimes can be heard in the chest, usually on the left side (the most common hernia is through the left-sided foramen of Bochdalek). Ventilation via a face mask may distend the stomach and further impair blood flow. Positive pressure ventilation with 100% oxygen should be given via an endotracheal tube. The normal lung is at risk of pneumothorax, and for this reason, high airway pressures should be avoided.

446. **The answer is A (1, 2, 3).** (Miller, 4/e. pp 1814, 2079.) Oxygen, parasympathetic stimulation, and acetylocloline all will close the ductus arteriosus in term animals. Prostaglandins are used to maintain the patency of the ductus arteriosus in situations where this is useful, for example, in a patient with pulmonary atresia.

447. **The answer is A (1, 2, 3).** (Stoelting, *Anesthesia and Co-Existing Disease,* 3/e. pp 43–45.) Attacks can occur spontaneously as well as with agitation. The etiology is thought to be infundibular spasm, which increases the right-to-left shunt. Squatting is thought to increase systemic vascular resistance, which reduces the right-to-left shunt and thereby improves circulation of blood through the lungs. Phenylephrine also increases systemic vascular resistance and reduces right-to-left shunt. Other treatments include hydration, pure oxygen, beta blockers, and morphine for sedation. Positive end-expiratory pressure and respiratory acidosis would both augment a right-to-left shunt and thereby worsen oxygenation.

448. **The answer is D (4).** (Barash, 3/e. pp 861–864.) Inhalational induction with halothane and nitrous oxide would be expected to be more prolonged because of the presence of a right-to-left shunt. Halothane is much more cardiodepressant in infants than in adults. The requirements for fentanyl in infants are extremely variable, but minimal cardiovascular effects are seen at 30 to 75 µg/kg.

449. **The answer is B (1, 3).** (Shnider, 3/e. pp 658–666, 694.) Uterine blood flow is insufficient in the setting of late decelerations and results in fetal hypoxia. Decelerations are due to either vagal discharge or direct myocardial depression, which results in bradycardia. Variable decelerations are thought to represent compression of the umbilical cord. When severe (i.e., fetal heart rates <60 to 70 beats per minutes lasting >60 s, especially when they persist for >30 min), they may indicate fetal compromise. A fetal scalp P_{O_2} of 25 mmHg is normal. A pH <7.20 is usually taken to indicate a distressed fetus.

450. **The answer is D (4).** (Stoelting, *Anesthesia and Co-Existing Disease,* 3/e. pp 579–580.) The neonatal airway anatomy differs from that of an adult in the following ways. The neonatal head and tongue are relatively larger than those of an adult. Neonates have smaller mouths than adults. The neonatal larynx has a large, floppy epiglottis, and the larynx is more anteriorly displaced than that of an adult. The narrowest portion of the neonatal larynx is subglottic at the cricoid cartilage. As a result of these characteristics, neonates may be more prone to upper airway obstruction caused by the tongue during mask ventilation. Also, an appropriately sized endotracheal tube that allows an air leak at 20 cmH$_2$O will prevent subglottic swelling.

451. **The answer is C (2, 4).** (Miller, 4/e. p 2090.) Clinical indicators of severe hypovolemia (15 percent volume depletion) include an entire cold extremity, absent posterior tibial pulse, capillary refill greater than 5 s, and mottled appearing skin.

452. **The answer is C (2, 4).** (Stoelting, *Anesthesia and Co-Existing Disease,* 3/e. pp 579–580.) The metabolic rate and resultant cardiac output of a newborn are double those of an adult. As a result, oxygen consumption in a newborn is double that of an adult (6 mL/kg/min versus 3 mL/kg/min), as is carbon dioxide production. To supply an appropriate amount of oxygen and prevent respiratory acidosis, minute ventilation is doubled in newborns compared with adults. Tidal volumes are the same in newborns and adults on a basis of milliliters per kilogram, but the respiratory rate is doubled in a newborn compared with an adult.

453. **The answer is E (all).** (Miller, 4/e. 1829–1830.) All of the above are major differences between adult and pediatric CPB.

454. **The answer is C (2, 4).** (Miller, 4/e. pp 2088–2090.) Guidelines for sodium bicarbonate include pH less than 7.0 and Pa$_{CO_2}$ less than 35 mmHg. Intraventricular hemorrhage may be secondary to increased volume or the increased CO$_2$ produced. Sodium bicarbonate will ultimately be converted to CO$_2$ and further exacerbate the respiratory acidosis. It also may interfere with myocardial function.

455. **The answer is A (1, 2, 3).** (Barash, 3/e. p 1110.) Patients with pyloric stenosis have persistent vomiting with loss of gastric HCl; a hypokalemic, hypochloremic metabolic alkalosis; dehydration; and compensatory respiratory acidosis.

456. **The answer is A (1, 2, 3).** (Barash, 3/e. p 931.) The patient has a potential full stomach (filled with blood), so that the airway needs to be quickly secured, and the patient may be severely hypovolemic from bleeding, which can be copious and unrecognized because much of it may be swallowed. Furthermore, the patient should have an intravenous line in place before induction. These are all reasons why an inhalational induction is a poor choice. An intravenous induction that uses agents that will support the circulation is indicated. A rapid sequence induction is needed. Succinylcholine is still considered the muscle relaxant of choice to achieve rapid paralysis. The risks of masseter spasm and malignant hyperthermia, while present, are small.

457. **The answer is C (2, 4).** (Miller, 4/e. p 2118.) Pyloric stenosis is not a surgical emergency. Dehydration and metabolic disturbances, specifically a hypochloremic, hypokalemic, metabolic alkalosis, should be corrected first. These patients present usually between 3 and 6 weeks of age and should have full stomach precautions.

458. **The answer is D (4).** (Miller, 4/e. p 2462.) Although rare at the extremes of age, epiglottitis can affect patients of any age. It occurs mostly in children 4 to 6 years old. In children, the disease may progress rapidly to airway obstruction, and so prophylactic intubation is nearly universally recommended. Racemic epinephrine is not part of the therapy. Most cases are due to *H. influenzae,* and the new vaccine is expected to reduce the incidence of this disease.

459. **The answer is B (1, 3).** (Miller, 4/e. p 2099.) In an adult, the narrowest part of the trachea is at the glottic opening; in an infant, at the cricoid. Alveoli increase in size and number until 8 years of age and increase only in size afterward. Dead space ventilation is similar in adults and infants. Closing capacity is greater than FRC in infants, leading to airway closure with each breath.

460. **The answer is A (1, 2, 3).** (Miller, 4/e. pp 968–969.) Patients with Down's syndrome (trisomy 21) have a high incidence of congenital heart defects. They frequently also have upper and lower airway abnormalities. In addition, they may have atlanto-occipital instability (C1–C2). The previously reported sensitivity to atropine has been disproved.

461. **The answer is E (all).** (Miller, 4/e. pp 2100–2102.) All the above are correct.

462. **The answer is D (4).** (Miller, 4/e. pp 2119–2120.) Although the use of regional anesthesia has been advocated to reduce the incidence of postoperative apnea in premature infants less than 60 weeks of postconceptional age, unequivocal data based on prospective, randomized, blinded studies are still lacking.

OBSTETRICS

Directions: Each question below contains four suggested responses of which **one or more** is correct. Select

(A)	if	**1, 2, and 3**	are correct
(B)	if	**1 and 3**	are correct
(C)	if	**2 and 4**	are correct
(D)	if	**4**	is correct
(E)	if	**1, 2, 3, and 4**	are correct

463. Cardiovascular changes that occur in obstetric patients include

(1) an increase in cardiac output
(2) an increase in heart rate and stroke volume
(3) a decrease in systemic vascular resistance
(4) a decrease in intravascular fluid volume

464. In patients with preeclampsia

(1) therapeutic magnesium levels are between 10 and 15 meq/L
(2) decreased levels of thromboxane are thought to be a possible etiologic factor
(3) the central nervous system shows decreased excitability
(4) hypotonia in a neonate born to a preeclamptic patient may be due to high magnesium levels.

465. True statements concerning breech deliveries include which of the following?

    (1)   They are associated with increased maternal morbidity

    (2)   Neonatal morbidity and mortality are both increased

    (3)   Regional anesthesia is not associated with a higher incidence of perinatal morbidity or maternal complications in breech vaginal deliveries

    (4)   During a vaginal breech delivery in a parturient with an epidural catheter in place, if the head gets stuck after the body is delivered and the obstetrician asks for uterine relaxation, appropriate anesthetic management consists of quickly topping off the epidural with a fast-acting local anesthetic, such as chloroprocaine

466. Regarding anesthesia during the course of normal labor,

(1) in the first stage of labor, pain impulses from the cervix and uterus travel with sympathetic nerve fibers and enter the spinal cord at T7–T10

(2) pain during the second stage of labor is somatic and is due to stretching of the perineal tissues; pain pathways reside in the pudendal nerve at S2–S4

(3) the ideal anesthetic for first stage labor is a paracervical block, since it provides good cervical anesthesia and has minimal hemodynamic effects

(4) the likelihood of a postdural puncture headache is greater in parturients than in nonpregnant patients

467. Regarding anesthetics used for cesarean section,

(1) steroid-based muscle relaxants cross the placenta much less easily than do nonsteroid muscle relaxants

(2) neonatal depression is seen with a ketamine dose of 1.5 mg/kg

(3) propofol has been shown in several studies to cause more hypotension than thiopental does

(4) use of halothane or isoflurane has not been demonstrated to increase blood loss

468. True statements about maternal physiology include which of the following?

(1) Functional residual capacity decreases during pregnancy by about 20 percent owing to decreases in both the residual and the expiratory reserve volumes

(2) Autoregulation of uterine blood vessels maintains constant uterine blood flow between mean arterial pressures of 50 and 150

(3) During pregnancy, the cardiac output increases, the systemic vascular resistance decreases, and the blood pressure decreases

(4) Aortocaval compression by a gravid uterus can cause uteroplacental insufficiency; the parturient should have her uterus displaced to the right by placing a wedge under the left buttock

469. Regarding obstetric anesthesia during labor, true statements include

(1) epinephrine should not be used in the epidural "test" dose because it may reduce uterine blood flow

(2) diazepam, when used in small doses for labor, has no effect on fetal heart rate, fetal acid-base status, or Apgar scores

(3) ketamine should not be used during labor for analgesia because it can have profound respiratory effects in the neonate

(4) morphine is not used for relief of labor pain because it is thought to cause more respiratory depression in newborns than does meperidine (Demerol)

470. True statements about a term fetus include

    (1) a normal fetal heart rate is 120 to 160 beats per minute

    (2) a normal fetal arterial blood gas is pH = 7.30, $P_{CO_2} = 45$, and $P_{O_2} = 25$

    (3) late decelerations on fetal monitoring can be an ominous sign; they indicate fetal asphyxia

    (4) succinylcholine does not cross the placenta because of its high molecular weight

471. Diabetes mellitus and its effects on the fetus include a greater incidence of

    (1) pregnancy-induced hypertension

    (2) respiratory distress of the newborn

    (3) malpresentations

    (4) small size for gestational age

472. Neurologic effects of magnesium sulfate ($MgSO_4$) include

    (1) decreased irritability of the central nervous system

    (2) decreased release of acetylcholine at the motor end plate

    (3) reduced sensitivity to acetylcholine at the motor end plate

    (4) relaxant effect on uterine and vascular smooth muscle

473. True statements concerning magnesium sulfate toxicity include

    (1) sluggish deep tendon reflexes are seen

    (2) motor weakness is shown

    (3) drowsiness occurs

    (4) serum magnesium levels of 4 to 6 meq/L are seen

474. Signs leading to the diagnosis of preeclampsia include

    (1) proteinuria

    (2) hypertension

    (3) generalized edema

    (4) hyperglycemia

475. Cardiovascular changes that occur in toxemia of pregnancy include

    (1) hypovolemia

    (2) hypertension

    (3) increased systemic vascular resistance leading to left ventricular dysfunction

    (4) decreased sensitivity to catecholamines

476. Regarding obstetric complications,

    (1) placenta previa and a previous cesarean section increase the risk of placenta accreta

    (2) placental abruption is associated with multiplicity and maternal hypertension

    (3) Asherman syndrome is associated with placenta accreta

    (4) polyhydramnios, multiparity, and retained placenta are all associated with uterine atony

477. Considerations in the anesthetic management of a 34-year-old woman with preeclampsia include

    (1)   decreased FRC and increased O_2 consumption in a pregnant parturient may contribute to an increased risk of the development of hypoxemia

    (2)   gastric acid volume is larger and gastric emptying is slower than in a nonpregnant patient; therefore, there is an increased risk of gastric aspiration

    (3)   there is a decrease in the dose requirement for local anesthetics during epidural and spinal anesthesia and for inhaled agents during general anesthesia in a pregnant patient

    (4)   an increased requirement for muscle relaxants may be seen with patients on magnesium sulfate for the treatment of preeclampsia

478. Regarding fetal monitoring,

(1) early decelerations are associated with compression of the fetal head and fetal distress

(2) fetal distress is associated with minimum to absent beat-to-beat variability of the fetal heart rate

(3) variable decelerations are rare and are best treated by supplying oxygen to the parturient

(4) late decelerations are most likely due to uteroplacental insufficiency

479. Consequences of the supine hypotension syndrome include

(1) decreased venous return to the right heart that leads to hypotension in the mother

(2) obstruction of the vena cava by the uterus

(3) uteroplacental insufficiency

(4) seizures in the mother

480. Drugs sometimes used during pregnancy or delivery and their potential side effects include

(1) ergot drugs and hypertension

(2) terbutaline and pulmonary edema

(3) magnesium and potentiation of both nondepolarizing and depolarizing muscle relaxants

(4) ritodrine and hyperkalemia

481. Properties applicable to drugs that diffuse slowly across the placenta include

(1) low maternal protein binding

(2) low molecular weight

(3) high lipid solubility

(4) high degree of ionization

482. Anesthetic considerations in a patient coming for cervical cerclage include which of the following?

(1) Spinal anesthesia should not be used because of the risk of sudden acute hypotension and the chance of uteroplacental hypoperfusion

(2) If the procedure is performed early in pregnancy, nitrous oxide should be avoided because of its possible inhibitory effects on DNA synthesis and its association with spontaneous abortions

(3) Monitoring of fetal heart rate and uterine activity should be used in all such patients

(4) Benzodiazepines probably should be avoided because of their association with teratogenicity

483. Major considerations concerning nonobstetric surgery in a parturient include which of the following?

(1) Avoidance of teratogenic drugs

(2) Prevention of fetal hypoxia and acidosis

(3) Incidence of premature labor

(4) Performance of elective surgery early rather than late in the pregnancy

484. A 24-year-old woman in her third trimester of pregnancy presents for emergency appendectomy. Important considerations for her anesthetic management include

(1) increased risk for premature labor

(2) increased risk for aspiration pneumonitis

(3) hypotensive syndrome associated with the supine position

(4) congenital anomalies resulting from exposure to trace amounts of anesthetics

485. Possible reasons for a reduction in anesthetic dose requirements during lumbar epidural analgesia in pregnancy include

(1) distention of the epidural venous plexus

(2) a reduction in buffer capacity secondary to respiratory alkalosis

(3) increased sensitivity of nerves secondary to the effects of progesterone

(4) increased lumbar lordosis during pregnancy

OBSTETRICS

ANSWERS

463. **The answer is A (1, 2, 3).** (Stoelting, *Anesthesia and Co-Existing Disease,* 3/e. pp 539–540.) Cardiac output increases in obstetric patients by about 40 percent during the first trimester, and this is maintained throughout pregnancy. The factors that increase cardiac output include increases in heart rate, contractility, and stroke volume and a decrease in systemic vascular resistance. These changes probably are mediated by ovarian and placental hormones. Intravascular fluid volume increases by approximately 35 percent, plasma volume more so than erythrocyte volume, which leads to the anemia of pregnancy.

464. **The answer is D (4).** (Miller, 4/e. pp 2061–2063.) The therapeutic magnesium level in treating preeclampsia is 4 to 6 meq/L. Levels above 10 meq/L are associated with loss of deep tendon reflexes. High thromboxane levels are thought to be a possible cause of preeclampsia, and substances, such as aspirin, which decrease thromboxane levels also decrease the incidence of preeclampsia. The central nervous system is hyperexcitable in preeclampsia. High levels of magnesium in a neonate may cause hypotonia as well as respiratory depression and apnea.

465. **The answer is A (1, 2, 3).** (Shnider, 3/e. pp 297–301.) Complications of breech delivery include cervical laceration and perineal injury, peripartum hemorrhage, and retained placenta. The neonate has a greater risk of trauma, especially to the head, and a higher incidence of prolapsed umbilical cord. In the emergency situation described, rapid uterine and perineal relaxation are needed and general anesthesia should be induced to provide those conditions. Breech delivery with a well-functioning regional anesthetic may be attempted from the beginning, but this will not provide profound uterine relaxation if that is needed.

466. **The answer is C (2, 4).** (Stoelting, *Anesthesia and Co-Existing Disease,* 3/e. pp 550–551.) Pain fibers from the cervix and uterus enter the spinal cord at T10–L1. A high incidence of fetal bradycardia occurs after paracervical block, which probably is related to rapid intravascular absorption into this highly vascular area. The drug readily crosses the placenta to the fetus. Headaches can be reduced when small needles are used, but parturients are nonetheless at particularly high risk for this complication.

467. **The answer is C (2, 4).** (Miller, 4/e. pp 2059–2060.) Muscle relaxants are charged molecules which cross the placenta in clinically insignificant amounts. There is no difference between steroid and nonsteroid muscle relaxants. Neonatal depression is seen with ketamine doses in excess of 1 mg/kg. Propofol has not been shown to cause any more hypotension than thiopental does. While halothane and isoflurane decrease uterine tone, they have not been shown to increase blood loss.

468. **The answer is B (1, 3).** (Miller, 4/e. pp 2031–2035. Shnider, 3/e. pp 3–12, 23–24.) A lowered functional residual capacity, combined with an elevated metabolism, means a limited oxygen reserve during pregnancy and rapid desaturation during apnea. For these reasons, careful denitrogenation before the induction of general anesthesia is recommended. Uterine blood flow is not autoregulated; it is pressure-dependent. Hypotension results in decreased uteroplacental perfusion. Left uterine displacement should be maintained in the parturient as much as possible to avoid aortocaval compression. This is done with a wedge placed under the right buttock.

469. **The answer is D (4).** (Shnider, 3/e. pp 38–39, 116–119, 124–125, 128.) While its use is controversial, epidural epinephrine is an excellent indicator of intravascular absorption. While it may reduce uterine blood flow, this effect is not clinically significant in a healthy fetus. No adverse effects in the fetus or neonate have been shown, but diazepam reduces fetal beat-to-beat variability and thus may confuse assessment of fetal well-being. Ketamine may increase maternal blood pressure and cause amnesia in a parturient, but at low doses (10 to 15 mg at a time, less than 100 mg in 30 min) there are no ill effects on the fetus. The preference for meperidine over morphine in obstetrics was based on a single study from 1965, but this is the stated reason for the preference.

470. **The answer is A (1, 2, 3).** (Miller, 4/e. pp 2079–2081. Shnider, 3/e. pp 22, 662.) Late decelerations are most ominous when fetal heart rate variability is lost. When late decelerations occur, the anesthesiologist should deliver oxygen to the mother, ensure adequate blood pressure and treat with pressor agents if necessary, and ensure left uterine displacement positioning. Succinylcholine does not appreciably cross the placenta because of its high degree of ionization. The nondepolarizing muscle relaxants do not cross the placenta because of their high molecular weight.

471. **The answer is A (1, 2, 3).** (Stoelting, *Anesthesia and Co-Existing Disease,* 3/e. pp 564–565.) Parturients who are suffering from diabetes mellitus often have babies who are large for gestational age. This may lead to malpresentations or other difficulties during vaginal deliveries. There is also a greater incidence of uteroplacental insufficiency. For these and other reasons, these patients often undergo elective and emergency cesarean sections.

472. **The answer is E (all).** (Stoelting, *Anesthesia and Co-Existing Disease,* 3/e. pp 562–563.) Magnesium sulfate is a CNS depressant and has all the listed effects in a toxemic parturient. Relaxation of the uterus may help improve uterine blood flow.

473. **The answer is A (1, 2, 3).** (Stoelting, *Anesthesia and Co-Existing Disease,* 3/e. pp 562–563.) Serum magnesium levels of 4 to 6 meq/L are deemed therapeutic. When serum levels are higher, one will see signs of magnesium toxicity. When serum levels are > 10 to 15 meq/L, ventilatory and cardiac failure occur.

474. **The answer is A (1, 2, 3).** (Stoelting, *Anesthesia and Co-Existing Disease,* 3/e. p 561.) Preeclampsia is a syndrome that occurs after the 20th week of pregnancy. Diagnosis is made when the parturient has the following three signs and symptoms: blood pressure greater than 140/90, proteinuria with urine protein greater than 2 g/day, and generalized edema. Hyperglycemia is not one of the diagnostic signs.

475. **The answer is A (1, 2, 3).** (Stoelting, *Anesthesia and Co-Existing Disease,* 3/e. p 562.) Cardiovascular changes that occur in toxemia of pregnancy include the following: first, there is a volume contraction, which leads to decreased right heart filling; second, there can be a direct decrease of inotropicity in this disease process of which the etiology is unknown; third, there is an increase in systemic vascular resistance, which can further impair left ventricular function. The net result is a patient who has volume contraction with a greatly reduced cardiac output, poor left ventricular reserve, hypertension, and poor perfusion of vital organs.

476. **The answer is E (all).** (Miller, 4/e. pp 2064–5065. Stoelting, 3/e. pp 565–567.) Placenta previa is a major cause of obstetric hemorrhage and occurs in 1 percent of full-term pregnancies. It is characterized by painless vaginal bleeding which stops spontaneously. Placental abruption accounts for about 33 percent of third trimester hemorrhages and also is associated with uterine anomalies and compression of the inferior vena cava. Asherman syndrome, which is the eponym for traumatic intrauterine synechiae, is associated with placenta accreta. Multiple births and a large fetus are also associated with uterine atony.

477. **The answer is A (1, 2, 3).** (Miller, 4/e. pp 2031–2067.) Magnesium treatment will reduce the requirement for both depolarizing and nondepolarizing muscle relaxants.

478. **The answer is C (2, 4).** (Stoelting, 3/e. pp 569–570.) Early decelerations, while associated with fetal heart compression, are not associated with fetal distress. Normal fetal heart rate is between 120 and 160 beats per minute, with normal beat-to-beat variability being between 5 and 20 beats per minute. Variable decelerations are the most common fetal heart rate and are thought to be due to umbilical cord compression. While atropine diminishes the severity of the variable decelerations, enhanced maternal oxygen delivery has no effect. Late decelerations, due to uteroplacental insufficiency, are a sign of fetal distress.

479. **The answer is A (1, 2, 3).** (Stoelting, *Anesthesia and Co-Existing Disease,* 3/e. pp 539–540.) The supine hypotension syndrome occurs in approximately 10 percent of pregnant women in the third trimester. When a pregnant woman lies flat, the gravid uterus will compress the vena cava, leading to a decrease in blood return to the right heart and a decrease in cardiac output. This in turn leads to hypotension with nausea, vomiting, and decreased cerebration in the mother and signs of uteroplacental insufficiency in the fetus. The gravid uterus also may compress the aorta. This will cause no symptoms in the mother but will cause further uteroplacental insufficiency in the fetus.

480. **The answer is A (1, 2, 3).** (Shnider, 3/e. pp 143, 315–316, 345, 531.) Alpha agonists with ergot drugs is an especially dangerous combination that can result in severe hypertension. Beta-adrenergic therapy can cause elevated myocardial oxygen demands and increased chronotropy and inotropy, the result of which can be myocardial ischemia, dysrhythmias, and heart failure. Magnesium decreases the amount of acetylcholine released into the myoneural junction, decreases the sensitivity of the motor end plate to acetylcholine, and depresses excitability of the muscle membrane. All these effects cause potentiation of the muscle relaxants. Hypokalemia results from beta-adrenergic agents such as ritodrine.

481. **The answer is D (4).** (Miller, 4/e. pp 2039–2040.) Properties that lead to slow diffusion across the placenta include a high degree of protein binding in the mother, high molecular weight, a low lipid solubility, and ionization. Drug concentration is also important. The lower the concentration is, the less drug crosses the placenta.

482. **The answer is C (2, 4).** (Katz, 3/e. p 167. Shnider, 3/e. pp 266–270.) A saddle (low spinal) block provides good surgical anesthesia and is safe as long as normotension is maintained with volume or pressors or both. Apart from its effects on methionine synthetase and DNA synthesis, which are controversial, nitrous oxide has been associated with spontaneous abortions, and since these procedures are often done in the late first trimester and early second trimester, these issues must be given consideration. Some obstetricians maintain that changes in heart rate and uterine activity are uninterpretable in young fetuses and that in any event no obstetric intervention (such as C-section) should be pursued before a certain gestational age. Although the association is unsubstantiated, diazepam has been implicated in birth defects, and by extension, all benzodiazepines may best be avoided.

483. **The answer is A (1, 2, 3).** (Stoelting, *Anesthesia and Co-Existing Disease,* 3/e. pp 567–569.) Elective surgery should be postponed as long as possible, preferably until after delivery. When surgery is semielective, the surgery should be performed as late as possible in the pregnancy so that the fetus has a better chance of survival if there is a preterm labor that cannot be arrested.

484. **The answer is A (1, 2, 3).** (Miller, 4/e. pp 2065–2067.) There is no evidence that anesthetics are teratogenic. In any event, the most vulnerable period for potential teratogenic effects is usually the first trimester.

485. **The answer is A (1, 2, 3).** (Cousins, 2/e. p 611.) With distention of the epidural venous plexus at term, the epidural space is smaller, so that a given amount of local anesthetic will have greater spread. A reduction in buffer capacity secondary to respiratory alkalosis is used to explain spread of epidural analgesia early in pregnancy, when mechanical factors (e.g., distention of epidural veins) are less likely to play a role. Progesterone may increase the sensitivity of isolated nerves to local anesthetics.

REGIONAL ANESTHESIA

Directions: Each question below contains five suggested responses. Select the **one best** response to each question.

486. Refer to the diagram below. Correct placement of drug for a celiac plexus block is at

(A) A
(B) B
(C) C
(D) D
(E) E

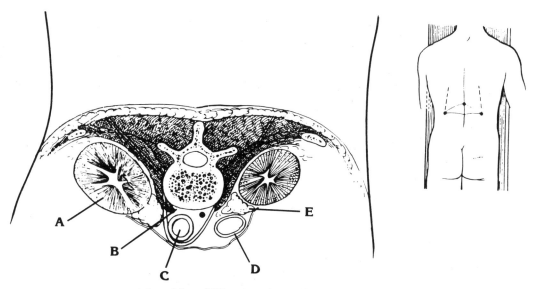

Adapted from Miller, *Anesthesia,* 4/e, with permission.

Questions 487–489

Refer to the diagram below.

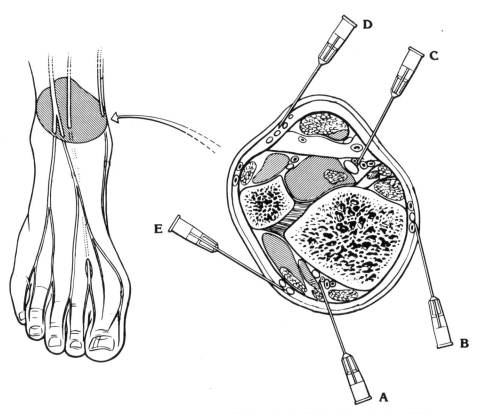

Adapted from Cousins MJ, Bridenbaugh PO (eds): *Neural Blockade in Clinical Anesthesia and Management of Pain,* 2/e, with permission.

487. The saphenous nerve is blocked at

    (A)   A
    (B)   B
    (C)   C
    (D)   D
    (E)   E

488. The deep peroneal nerve is blocked by needle placement at

    (A)   A
    (B)   B
    (C)   C
    (D)   D
    (E)   E

489. The sural nerve is blocked by needle placement at

  (A)   A
  (B)   B
  (C)   C
  (D)   D
  (E)   E

490. All the following statements are true EXCEPT

  (A)   nerve supply to the foot is derived mainly from branches of the sciatic nerve
  (B)   sensation to the sole of the foot is supplied mainly by the sural nerve
  (C)   the saphenous nerve is the only branch of the femoral nerve to supply sensation below the knee
  (D)   the dorsum of the foot is supplied by the deep peroneal and saphenous nerves
  (E)   all the nerves supplying sensation to the foot can be blocked at the ankle

Directions: Each question below contains four suggested responses of which **one or more** is correct. Select

(A)	if	**1, 2, and 3**	are correct
(B)	if	**1 and 3**	are correct
(C)	if	**2 and 4**	are correct
(D)	if	**4**	is correct
(E)	if	**1, 2, 3, and 4**	are correct

491. True statements regarding nerve transmission include

(1) spinal blockade is rapid and requires only a small dose of local anesthetic because the axons of these nerves lack surrounding fibrous tissue and fat so that local anesthetics can easily reach and penetrate them

(2) the main determinant of local anesthetic potency is lipid solubility

(3) the axons in large nerve trunks, such as those which innervate the limbs, are arranged so that outer fibers innervate proximal limb parts while inner fibers innervate distal limb parts

(4) pain is mediated by A delta fibers and C fibers, neither of which are myelinated

492. Regarding the development of the spinal cord and vertebral column,

(1) at birth the spinal cord terminates at L4

(2) at birth the dural sac terminates at S3–S4

(3) at birth lumbar lordosis and cervical flexure are absent

(4) myelinization, while not complete at birth, is greatest in the nerve trunks of the lower extremities

493. In performing an infraclavicular block,

(1) there is a decreased likelihood of pneumothorax

(2) a nerve stimulator is not necessary

(3) injection occurs at a level which blocks both musculocutaneous and axillary nerves

(4) the needle is advanced medially toward the C6 tubercle

494. True statements with respect to laryngeal innervation include

(1) two branches of the vagus nerve are entirely responsible for the motor and sensory innervation of the larynx

(2) the recurrent laryngeal nerve innervates all the motor supply of the larynx

(3) the superior laryngeal nerve innervates all the sensory supply of the larynx above the cords

(4) the motor innervation for the cricothyroid muscle is dually supplied by the superior laryngeal nerve and the recurrent laryngeal nerve

495. Complications after retrobulbar block include

(1) hemorrhage

(2) vagal stimulation

(3) direct trauma to the eye

(4) brainstem anesthesia

496. Accurate statements about the cervical plexus include

(1) blockade of the superficial cervical plexus will anesthetize the cutaneous nerves of the neck and includes branches from C1–C4
(2) the deep cervical plexus innervates the neck muscles
(3) by blocking the cervical plexus (both deep and superficial), one can perform surgery on the thyroid, trachea, and carotid artery
(4) phrenic nerve paralysis is not a risk in performing a cervical plexus block

497. True statements about airway structures include

(1) the fifth cranial nerve (trigeminal) provides sensory innervation to the posterior two-thirds of the tongue
(2) 4% cocaine can be used safely as a topical anesthetic and vasoconstrictor for the nasal passages as long as the total dose does not exceed 5 mg/kg
(3) the posterior cricoarytenoid muscle is innervated by the superior laryngeal nerve
(4) the vocal cords receive motor innervation from the vagus nerve

498. Complications of a stellate ganglion block include

(1) block of the recurrent laryngeal nerve
(2) spinal injection
(3) intravascular injection
(4) block of the superior laryngeal nerve

499. Which of the following signs would suggest a successful stellate ganglion block?

(1) Cooler skin temperature on the contralateral side
(2) Nasal stuffiness
(3) Horner's syndrome
(4) Numbness of the skin in the neck area

500. Landmarks for a stellate ganglion block include

(1) the sternocleidomastoid muscle
(2) the trachea
(3) Chassaignac's tubercle
(4) the thyroid cartilage

501. Complications of the interscalene approach to the brachial plexus include

(1) phrenic nerve blockade
(2) vagus nerve damage
(3) intrathecal injection
(4) puncture of the aortic root with the block needle

502. A Bier block in the upper extremity is correctly characterized by which of the following statements?

(1) There is a high risk of systemic toxicity because of the large dose of local anesthetic that must be used
(2) The double-tourniquet technique can actually prolong the effectiveness of the block
(3) Before placing the block, exsanguination of the upper extremity is necessary for complete effectiveness
(4) An advantage of this block is its long duration of action, which often outlasts surgery and gives postoperative pain relief

SUMMARY OF DIRECTIONS

A	B	C	D	E
1,2,3 only	1,3 only	2,4 only	4 only	All are correct

503. True statements about nerves to the hand include

   (1) the median nerve arises from both the lateral and the medial cords of the brachial plexus

   (2) the ulnar nerve arises solely from the lateral cord of the brachial plexus

   (3) pronation of the wrist is a function of the median nerve

   (4) the fingernail of the middle finger receives sensory innervation from the radial nerve

504. True statements about nerve supply to the hand include which of the following?

   (1) Supination of the hand is a function of the radial nerve

   (2) Loss of ability to touch thumb to fifth finger after elbow injury is most likely due to injury to the nerve located just medial to the brachial artery in the antecubital fossa

   (3) Sensory loss of the fifth finger attributable to nerve root injury is most likely due to a C8 lesion, a T1 lesion, or both

   (4) Isolated inability to flex the elbow with sensory deficits along the lateral aspect of the forearm after an injury to the axilla suggests a lesion of the lateral cord of the brachial plexus

505. Possible complications associated with intercostal nerve blocks include

   (1) pneumothorax

   (2) convulsions from systemic absorption of local anesthetics

   (3) respiratory insufficiency

   (4) subarachnoid injection of local anesthetics

506. True statements about blocking the brachial plexus in the axilla include

   (1) the major complication is a pneumothorax

   (2) it produces good anesthesia for shoulder surgery

   (3) the musculocutaneous nerve is reliably blocked with this approach

   (4) radial nerve paresthesias usually are elicited deep to the axillary artery

507. True statements about nerve supply to the lower extremity include

   (1) the femoral nerve arises from the L5, S1, and S2 nerve roots

   (2) adequate anesthesia for an above-the-knee amputation requires blockade of the femoral, sciatic, obturator, and lateral femoral cutaneous nerves

   (3) the posterior tibial nerve can be blocked at the ankle joint just lateral to the lateral malleolus

   (4) the inner aspect of the large toe is innervated by the deep peroneal nerve, which can be blocked between the tendons of the extensor hallucis longus and the anterior tibial muscle

508. When one is performing a peripheral nerve block for knee arthroscopy, it is necessary to block the

(1) femoral nerve
(2) lateral femoral cutaneous nerve
(3) obturator nerve
(4) superficial peroneal nerve

509. Spinal blockade is correctly characterized by which of the following statements?

(1) Arterial vasodilation is the main mechanism for the decrease in blood pressure seen with a T10 spinal blockade
(2) The arterial blood gas (ABG) of a nonsedated patient breathing quietly after spinal blockade with a T4 sensory level will show a mild respiratory acidosis with normal oxygenation
(3) Numbness of the little finger after spinal blockade represents an approximately T4 sensory level
(4) With a T4 sensory level after spinal blockade, bradycardia may be seen because the sympathetic block is approximately two spinal segments higher than the sensory block

510. True statements regarding spinal blockade include which of the following?

(1) With spinal anesthesia, neural blockade is due primarily to penetration of local anesthetic into the spinal cord
(2) Precipitous hypotension during high spinal anesthesia in a normovolemic patient is primarily due to a profound reduction in systemic vascular resistance
(3) Elimination of local anesthetics from the subarachnoid space primarily involves their metabolism in cerebrospinal fluid
(4) Zones of differential blockade (sensory, motor, sympathetic) can be demonstrated at the cephalic end of a spinal block; these zones correspond to regions of differing concentrations of local anesthetic solution in the cerebrospinal fluid

511. Regarding the anatomy of the vertebral column,

(1) the ligament first pierced by an epidural needle using the midline approach is the posterior longitudinal ligament
(2) the epidural space at L2 in an adult is 1 to 2 mm in width
(3) the cephalic limit of the epidural space is C1
(4) damage to the radicularis magna (artery of Adamkiewicz) is a potential complication of a properly performed spinal block

512. Factors that probably are significantly related to the height of spinal anesthetic block include

  (1) addition of a vasoconstrictor
  (2) gender of patient
  (3) increased intraabdominal pressure
  (4) baricity of solution injected

513. True statements about local anesthetic solutions for spinal anesthesia include which of the following?

  (1) Among lidocaine, bupivacaine, and tetracaine, the local anesthetic most likely to demonstrate a substantially prolonged duration of spinal anesthesia with the addition of 0.2 to 0.3 mg of epinephrine is tetracaine
  (2) The specific gravity of cerebrospinal fluid is approximately 1.006
  (3) The baricity of local anesthetic solution for spinal anesthesia is the ratio of the density of the solution divided by that of cerebrospinal fluid
  (4) A local anesthetic solution with a baricity of 1.002 is hyperbaric

SUMMARY OF DIRECTIONS

A	B	C	D	E
1,2,3 only	1,3 only	2,4 only	4 only	All are correct

514. Addition of epinephrine to 0.5% bupivacaine for epidural anesthesia

(1) speeds the onset of block
(2) affects the lipophilicity of bupivacaine
(3) decreases the vascular absorption of drug
(4) has a minimal effect on the duration of block

515. The incidence of headache after dural puncture

(1) is higher in females than in males
(2) is near zero in patients older than 50 years of age
(3) is related to the gauge of the spinal needle
(4) is lower when a higher glucose concentration is used in the local anesthetic solution

516. Complications associated with intraspinal narcotics include

(1) respiratory depression
(2) pruritus
(3) urinary retention
(4) motor blockade

517. Nausea and vomiting associated with intraspinal narcotics are due to

(1) systemic absorption
(2) allergic reactions to the drug
(3) local effect on opioid receptors
(4) rostral spread to the chemoreceptor trigger zone

518. True statements about the epidural space include

(1) the epidural space is a potential space that surrounds the dura mater
(2) the epidural space contains nerve roots, fat, and blood vessels
(3) the epidural space extends from the foramen magnum to the sacral hiatus
(4) the posterior border of the epidural space is the ligamentum flavum

519. Physiologic differences between spinal block and epidural block include

(1) level of sympathectomy with a given sensory blockade
(2) effects on the respiratory system
(3) systemic blood levels of drug
(4) effects on renal function

520. Complications of epidural blockade include

(1) intravascular injection
(2) subarachnoid injection
(3) neurologic injury
(4) epidural hematoma

521. Correct statements concerning celiac plexus block include

(1) it is useful for controlling the pain associated with cancer of the upper abdominal viscera
(2) skin numbness in a T5–T10 dermatomal distribution is a sign of a successful block
(3) possible complications include subarachnoid and intraaortic injections
(4) the anterior, subxiphoid, approach is safest, since it avoids potential injury to retroperitoneal structures

522. Nerves anesthetized in the lumbar
plexus block include the

(1)   femoral nerve
(2)   obturator nerve
(3)   lateral femoral cutaneous nerve
(4)   sciatic nerve

REGIONAL
ANESTHESIA

A N S W E R S

486. The answer is B. (Miller, 4/e. pp 1560–1561.) The celiac plexus is located by walking a needle off the body of T12 or L1 on the left side of the patient. Pulsations through the needle signify the proximity of the aorta and correct placement. A needle is placed on the right side to a similar depth. Drug is injected after aspiration for blood or CSF. In the diagram below, *A* is the aorta and *IVC* is the inferior vena cava.

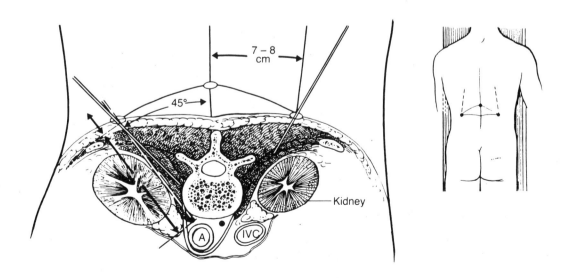

487–489. The answers are: 487-B, 488-A, 489-D. (Barash, 3/e. pp 695–696.) The saphenous nerve innervates an area along the medial aspect of the foot. It is located near the saphenous vein, anterior to the medial malleolus.

The deep peroneal nerve innervates the dorsum of the foot. It is located between the tendons of the anterior tibial and extensor hallucis longus muscles. These landmarks are more visible when the patient dorsiflexes the foot.

The sural nerve is blocked by infiltration between the lateral malleolus and the Achilles tendon. This provides anesthesia of the lateral foot and the lateral proximal sole of the foot.

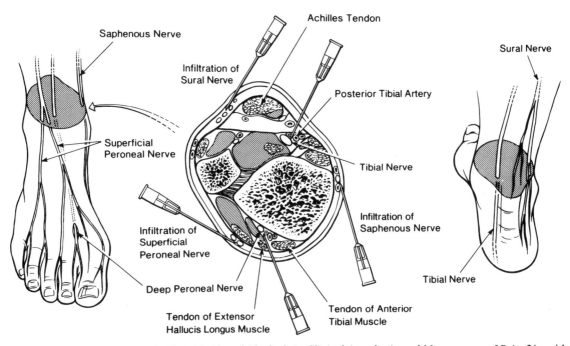

From Cousins MJ, Bridenbaugh PO (eds): *Neural Blockade in Clinical Anesthesia and Management of Pain,* 2/e, with permission.

490. The answer is B. (Miller, 4/e. pp 1552–1553.) The posterior tibial nerve is the major source of innervation to the sole of the foot.

491. The answer is A (1, 2, 3) (Cousins, 2/e. pp 35, 38, 39, 111.) Many factors determine how quickly local anesthetics penetrate and block individual nerves; the tissue barriers between local anesthetic deposition and axoplasm of the nerve are an important factor. Local anesthetics gradually penetrate from the outer to the inner nerve trunks. This explains why anesthesia of a limb spreads in a proximal to distal direction. C fibers are unmyelinated and conduct pain-related impulses slowly, while A delta fibers are myelinated and convey signals rapidly. C fibers also mediate postganglionic autonomic nerve transmission.

492. **The answer is A (1, 2, 3).** (Miller, 4/e. pp 1565–1566.) Contemplation of centroneuraxis anesthesia must take into account the differences which exist in the pediatric population. By age 2 the level of the dural sac and spinal cord approaches adult levels, but at birth these structures terminate farther caudad. Lumbar lordosis and cervical flexure develop in response to sitting and sustaining head position, respectively, abilities that are absent at birth. Myelinization is not complete at birth but proceeds in a cephalad-to-caudad direction with the nerve trunks of the lower extremities being myelinated later.

493. **The answer is B (1, 3).** (Miller, 4/e. p 1542.) The decreased likelihood of pneumothorax and blocking of the axillary and musculocutaneous nerves in one injection are two of the infraclavicular block's purported advantages. The frequent absence of any vascular landmarks, except in a very thin person, makes the nerve stimulator a requirement. The needle is advanced laterally in a line from the C6 tubercle to the axillary artery palpated in the axilla, with the insertion point being 2 cm below the mid-clavicle.

494. **The answer is B (1, 3).** (Miller, 4/e. p 1404.) Two branches of the vagus nerve are entirely responsible for the motor and sensory innervation of the larynx: the superior and the recurrent laryngeal nerves. The superior laryngeal nerve innervates all the sensory supply of the larynx above the cords and all the motor supply of the cricothyroid muscle.

495. **The answer is E (all).** (Miller, 4/e. p 1558.) Retrobulbar blocks are extremely safe, but complications can occur. Hemorrhage occurs in 1 in 700 blocks and is treated with gentle pressure for 20 to 30 min. The oculocardiac reflex manifests as bradycardia and other signs of vagal stimulation. Atropine can be given to reduce these effects. Direct trauma to the eye and brainstem anesthesia are very rare but can be minimized by paying strict attention to technique and not penetrating too deeply into the orbit.

496. **The answer is A (1, 2, 3).** (Miller, 4/e. pp 1555–1556.) Deep cervical plexus block is associated with several possible complications. The phrenic or superior laryngeal nerves can be paralyzed. Intravascular (especially vertebral artery), epidural, or subarachnoid injections are possible complications of this block. Complications of the superficial plexus block are fewer and less dangerous; the most common complication is blockade of the spinal accessory nerve, which causes paralysis of the trapezius muscle.

497. **The answer is D (4).** (Miller, 4/e. pp 2184, 2193.) The anterior two-thirds of the tongue is innervated by the trigeminal nerve. The posterior third of the tongue receives sensory innervation from the ninth cranial nerve (glossopharyngeal). Cocaine is effective, but absorption from the nasal mucosa is high and the dose should not exceed 1.5 mg/kg to avoid local anesthetic toxicity. The posterior cricoarytenoid muscle is innervated by the recurrent laryngeal nerve (as are all intrinsic muscles of the larynx except for the cricothyroid muscle). It is the only abductor of the vocal cords, so that injury or nerve blockade with local anesthetics will cause the ipsilateral vocal cord to assume a more midline position, resulting in glottic narrowing and hoarseness. The recurrent laryngeal nerve and possibly the superior laryngeal nerve, both of which are branches of the vagus, supply the vocal cords with motor innervation.

498. **The answer is A (1, 2, 3).** (Miller, 4/e. p 1559.) The superior laryngeal nerve is remote from the injection site of a stellate ganglion block. All the other complications, however, have been reported. Seizures and cardiac dysrhythmias and cardiac collapse can result from intravascular injection. Of special concern is the close proximity of the vertebral artery to the injection site. Vertebral artery injection of only a tiny dose of local anesthetic will result in instantaneous convulsions, as toxic cerebral concentrations are rapidly reached. Subarachnoid and brachial plexus blocks also can occur.

499. **The answer is A (1, 2, 3).** (Miller, 4/e. p 1559.) Signs of successful stellate ganglion block include warmer skin on the side of block, Horner's syndrome, nasal stuffiness, injection of conjunctiva, and vasodilation.

500. **The answer is A (1, 2, 3).** (Miller, 4/e. p 1559.) Horner's syndrome [enophthalmos (sinking of the eyeball), miosis, and ptosis], anhidrosis, and conjunctival injection are signs of a successful stellate ganglion block. The first three listed landmarks are appropriate for this block.

501. **The answer is A (1, 2, 3).** (Miller, 4/e. p 1536.) When one is performing a brachial plexus block via the interscalene approach, the landmarks for needle insertion are as follows: the nerve trunks are at the level of the cricoid cartilage, which is at C6 and posterior to the sternocleidomastoid muscle between the anterior and medial scalene muscles. The root of the aorta lies in the midline below the manubrium; therefore, the block needle should not be near the aorta. However, vertebral artery and carotid artery injections have been described with the interscalene approach.

502. **The answer is A (1, 2, 3).** (Miller, 4/e. p 1545.) One of the disadvantages of a Bier block is that it is of short duration (45 to 60 min). Exsanguination of the limb is necessary to keep the local anesthetic confined to the upper extremity. As soon as circulation returns, the block is over, since the local anesthetic is washed away. Because a high dose of anesthetic is administered, there is a high risk of systemic toxicity if the block is not placed properly. Tourniquets prevent the large dose from entering the circulation too quickly, and 25 to 35 min after placement is usually enough time for drug levels to fall below those of systemic toxicity. The double tourniquet prolongs the block by prolonging the time during which patients can endure the tourniquet pain. Initially, only the proximal tourniquet is inflated. When pain is felt here, the distal tourniquet is inflated over an area of anesthetized skin and the proximal tourniquet is deflated.

503. **The answer is B (1, 3).** (Wedel, p 257. Cousins, 2/e. p 406.) The ulnar nerve arises solely from the medial cord. Sensory innervation of the fingernail of the middle finger is from the median nerve.

504. **The answer is B (1, 3).** (Wedel, pp 258, 267. Cousins, 2/e. p 406.) The ability to touch the thumb to the fifth finger is mediated by the ulnar nerve, which at the elbow is posterior to the medial epicondyle of the humerus. The median nerve is just medial to the brachial artery at the elbow. The motor and sensory dysfunctions described in choice 4 are both attributable to damage of the musculocutaneous nerve, which is a terminal branch of the lateral cord of the brachial plexus.

505. **The answer is A (1, 2, 3).** (Miller, 4/e. p 1559.) Pneumothorax and problems from systemic absorption of local anesthetics are the most common complications. In patients with severe pulmonary disease who rely on their intercostal muscles, respiratory insufficiency may result after bilateral multiple blocks.

506. **The answer is D (4).** (Miller, 4/e. p 1540.) The axillary approach to the brachial plexus avoids a pneumothorax. Good anesthesia is obtained for the lower arm but not for upper arm or shoulder surgery. The musculocutaneous nerve is often not in the axillary sheath, and so it is not reliably blocked. Injecting local anesthetic into the coracobrachialis muscle will anesthetize this nerve.

507. **The answer is C (2, 4).** (Miller, 4/e. pp 1546, 1552–1553.) The femoral nerve arises from the posterior divisions of the L2, L3, and L4 nerve roots. The posterior tibial nerve is a branch of the sciatic nerve and is located at the ankle just lateral to the medial malleolus.

508. **The answer is A (1, 2, 3).** (Miller, 4/e. pp 1547–1548.) The femoral nerve innervates the anterior and medial thigh and knee. The lateral femoral cutaneous nerve innervates the lateral thigh, and blockade of all three nerves is necessary to block tourniquet pain. The obturator nerve innervates the medial thigh area. The superficial peroneal nerve is one of the terminal branches of the sciatic nerve; its sensory distribution is below the knee.

509. **The answer is D (4).** (Barash, 3/e. pp 648, 661–663.) Venodilation with pooling of blood in the lower extremities and decreased venous return to the heart with decreased cardiac output are responsible for the hypotension seen with a T10 spinal level. A T4 renders a patient unable to cough and clear secretions, but the resting ABG will be normal. Numbness of the little finger represents a C8 level.

510. **The answer is D (4).** (Cousins, 2/e. pp 227–229, 231.) Although penetration of local anesthetic into the spinal cord occurs to some extent, neural blockade is primarily due to the action of local anesthetics on nerve roots and in dorsal root ganglia. Systemic vascular resistance is modestly altered; the mechanism of hypotension involves reduction in cardiac output resulting from reductions in preload. Local anesthetics are eliminated by vascular absorption in the subarachnoid and epidural spaces, followed by metabolism of the esters in the bloodstream or that of amides in the liver. Sympathetic preganglionic nerves are the most easily blocked so that dilute local anesthetic concentrations, present at the farthest point of spread from the injection site, block these nerves but not the more resistant somatic sensory or motor nerves. The A alpha motor neurons are the most difficult to block, and so the area of motor blockade has the most limited cephalic spread.

511. **The answer is D (4).** (Cousins, 2/e. p 220. Miller, 4/e. pp 1507–1510.) The first ligament encountered is the supraspinous (connecting the tips of the spinous processes to each other), then the interspinous ligament (connecting the bodies of the spinous processes to each other), and finally the ligamentum flavum. The posterior longitudinal ligament extends along the posterior surfaces of the vertebral bodies. The epidural space is widest at L2: 5 to 6 mm in an average adult. The caudal limit of the epidural space is the sacral hiatus; the cephalic limit is the foramen magnum. The radicularis magna, which is the major feeder artery to the anterior spinal artery at the level of the lumbosacral spinal cord, enters the spinal canal through an intervertebral foramen anywhere between T8 and L3 and therefore can be damaged by a spinal needle. This can result in ischemia of the lumbar region of the spinal cord.

512. **The answer is D (4).** (Miller, 4/e. p 152.) Though many factors—such as age, height, gender, increased intraabdominal pressure, vasoconstrictors, barbotage, and the Valsalva maneuver—have all been implicated in raising the level of a spinal anesthetic, they probably have little, if any, effect at all. Patient position, dose, and the baricity of the solution are the only characteristics known to significantly affect the level.

513. **The answer is E (all).** (Cousins, 2/e. pp 222, 223, 225.) The duration of action of lidocaine and bupivacaine is affected by epinephrine much less than is that of tetracaine. Baricity is defined correctly in choice 3. It follows that the baricity of cerebrospinal fluid is 1.000 and that values above 1.001 or below 0.999 will render a solution, respectively, hyper- or hypobaric.

514. **The answer is D (4).** (Miller, 3/e. p 452.) Addition of vasoconstrictors to 0.5% bupivacaine for epidural anesthesia has virtually no effect on the duration of action or any other characteristic of the drug. This is probably the case because bupivacaine is very lipophilic and is quickly absorbed into local fat tissue. From there it is slowly released and causes a prolonged block. Epinephrine does not affect this lipophilic quality. However, blocks using dilute solutions, such as 0.25% bupivacaine, may be prolonged with epinephrine.

515. **The answer is B (1, 3).** (Miller, 4/e. pp 1520–1521.) Headache after dural puncture occurs less frequently with increasing age, but it is still a potential problem in elderly patients. The incidence of this headache increases with increasing glucose concentration in the local anesthetic solution.

516. **The answer is A (1, 2, 3).** (Miller, 4/e. pp 2334–2336.) Motor blockade is not associated with the use of intraspinal narcotics. The other three effects are commonly seen, with delayed respiratory depression being the most problematic. All these side effects can be alleviated by naloxone, but at the risk of losing analgesia.

517. **The answer is D (4).** (Miller, 4/e. p 2336.) Rostral spread to the chemoreceptor trigger zone is thought to be the major cause of nausea and vomiting. The more hydrophilic drugs, such as morphine, are more likely to be associated with this problem than are lipophilic drugs, such as fentanyl, because hydrophilic drugs will spread rostrally without being locally absorbed.

518. **The answer is E (all).** (Miller, 4/e. p 1507.) The epidural space surrounds the dura mater on all sides from the foramen magnum to the sacral hiatus. Posteriorly, the ligamentum flavum serves as a landmark for approaching the epidural space.

519. **The answer is B (1, 3).** (Miller, 4/e. pp 1511–1512.) Subarachnoid block usually will give a sympathetic block between two and six dermatomes higher than the sensory block, whereas epidural sympathetic block is at the same dermatomal level as the sensory block. There are two reasons for higher serum drug levels with epidural blocks. First, the greater vascularity of the epidural space results in more intravascular drug absorption; second, large volumes of drug are required for epidural blockade, which makes it easier to achieve toxic levels. The effect of both blocks on the respiratory system is minimal and depends on the level of motor and sensory block achieved. Renal function is affected by mean arterial pressure rather than by the block itself.

520. **The answer is E (all).** (Miller, 4/e. pp 1527–1528.) All the listed problems are possible with epidural placement. Aspiration of the needle or catheter to check for blood or CSF usually reduces the chance of subarachnoid or intravascular injection. Epinephrine-containing solutions are helpful in determining intravascular injection but are not always reliable, especially in patients on beta blockers. Neurologic injury is exceedingly rare and is most likely due to epidural hematoma formation with compression of the spinal cord. Direct nerve injury is rare with this technique because nerves do not traverse the epidural space posteriorly, where the needle is placed. Rapid evaluation of any possible neurologic injury after an epidural block is most important because early diagnosis and drainage of an epidural hematoma may prevent permanent nerve damage.

521. **The answer is B (1, 3).** (Miller, 4/e. pp 1560–1561.) The celiac plexus innervates the viscera of the upper abdomen. Neurolytic block gives excellent relief of cancer pain from the pancreas, stomach, and liver. However, this block wears off with time, and so it is less useful for chronic conditions associated with long life spans, such as pancreatitis. Because the vasoconstrictor fibers of the viscera are also blocked, postural hypotension is a common problem. Subarachnoid and intraaortic injections are both possible. Fluoroscopic confirmation of needle placement is recommended before neurolytic blocks are performed. Large volumes of drugs are necessary for celiac plexus block, and so spread to lumbar nerves is a risk. The celiac plexus contains autonomic fibers derived from T5–T12 to the abdominal viscera; it contains no somatic fibers, and so skin numbness is not expected. The posterior approach is the only recommended way to perform the block. While it does invade the retroperitoneal space, it is far safer than a transabdominal approach.

522. **The answer is A (1, 2, 3).** (Miller, 4/e. pp 1546–1547.) The block is also known as the "three-in-one" block. The sciatic nerve is formed by the L4–S3 nerve roots and is not blocked in this approach.

POSITIONING AND SAFETY

Directions: Each question below contains five suggested responses. Select the **one best** response to each question.

523. Regarding electrical power in the operating room (OR), all the following are true EXCEPT

- (A) in an isolated system the electrical power is ungrounded
- (B) the line isolation monitor (LIM) continuously monitors electrical power to ensure that it is isolated from the ground
- (C) plugging a short-circuited piece of equipment into an isolated power system will result in its inactivation
- (D) the use of an electrosurgical unit ("Bovie") does not require a patient to be grounded
- (E) ventricular fibrillation may be caused by as little as 0.1 mA in microshock

524. All the following statements are true EXCEPT

- (A) ventricular fibrillation can be caused by currents below the level of human perception in a patient with a PA catheter
- (B) equipment ground wires provide the major source of protection from microshock
- (C) Ohm's law states that current (I) is equal to the product of resistance (R) and electromotive force (V)
- (D) a dry ground pad on a patient can result in skin burns
- (E) from the point of view of electrical safety, bipolar is safer than unipolar electrosurgery

525. Universal precautions for handling blood and body fluids as put forth by the Centers for Disease Control (CDC) apply to

(A) only patients suspected of having communicable diseases

(B) body fluids containing visible blood but not to clear cerebrospinal fluid

(C) use of appropriate barriers for the procedure being performed, such as gloves or masks, although protective eyewear is never indicated

(D) handling of pleural fluid or synovial fluid but not to tears or sweat

(E) handling of saliva and sputum, since HIV infection is readily transmitted via these routes

526. In comparing two different measurements, what percentage of the data pairs will fall within two standard deviations of the differences, assuming a normal distribution?

(A) 50 percent
(B) 68 percent
(C) 87 percent
(D) 95 percent
(E) 99 percent

527. All the following statements about addiction within the profession of anesthesiology are true EXCEPT

(A) several retrospective surveys show that the prevalence of chemical dependence is 1 to 2 percent

(B) sufentanil is considered to have less addictive potential than meperidine

(C) chemically dependent physicians usually are not identified until late stages of the disease

(D) strict methods of dispensing addictive drugs to members of anesthesiology departments have been shown to be an important deterrent to drug addiction

(E) recovering addicts are allowed to take the ABA written and oral board examinations

Directions: Each question below contains four suggested responses of which **one or more** is correct. Select

(A)	if	**1, 2, and 3**	are correct
(B)	if	**1 and 3**	are correct
(C)	if	**2 and 4**	are correct
(D)	if	**4**	is correct
(E)	if	**1, 2, 3, and 4**	are correct

528. True statements pertaining to the lateral decubitus position include

(1) in an awake, spontaneously breathing patient, ventilation and perfusion are greatest in the dependent lung

(2) in an awake, spontaneously breathing patient in this position, the ventilation-perfusion (V/Q) ratio is greatest in the nondependent lung

(3) ventilation-perfusion mismatch is greater in an anesthetized than in an awake patient in this position

(4) in comparison with an awake patient in the lateral decubitus position, an anesthetized, paralyzed, and mechanically ventilated patient has relatively more ventilation to the dependent lung

529. Correct statements about nerve injuries caused by malpositioning of the patient include

(1) sciatic nerve injuries are the most common

(2) stirrups used in the lithotomy position can put pressure on the saphenous nerve and lead to inability to plantarflex the foot postoperatively

(3) when placed on armboards, the arms may be safely abducted to 120° without causing brachial plexus injury

(4) an anesthetized patient is likely to have exaggerated changes in blood pressure in response to changes in body position

530. Injuries during procedures are accurately characterized by which of the following descriptions?

(1) Hypesthesia of the front and lateral aspects of the thigh after a difficult forceps delivery is most likely due to pressure of the forceps on the obturator nerve

(2) With arms on armboards, hands should be pronated with elbows well padded to avoid ulnar nerve injury

(3) Alopecia after long operations may occur and is most likely due to the inhibitory influence of the halogenated inhalational anesthetics on hair growth

(4) Trendelenburg position is likely to produce ventilation-perfusion inequalities

531. True statements regarding temperature regulation include

(1) general anesthesia does not markedly alter the body temperature at which vasoconstriction occurs to conserve body heat

(2) mild hypothermia (34°C) appears to have a protective effect against brain ischemia, wound infection, and blood coagulation

(3) the rapid reduction of core body temperature that develops immediately after induction of general anesthesia is primarily due to evaporation of surgical skin preparation solutions and is easily preventable

(4) airway warming and humidification do not have a dramatic effect on maintenance of normal body temperature

SUMMARY OF DIRECTIONS

A	B	C	D	E
1,2,3 only	1,3 only	2,4 only	4 only	All are correct

532. Intraoperative hypothermia may cause

(1) ST elevations known as *Ashman waves*

(2) an inability to antagonize nondepolarizing muscle relaxants with anticholinesterase drugs

(3) hyperventilation in newborns

(4) a left-shifted oxyhemoglobin dissociation curve

533. Regarding statistical methods,

(1) the Student's t test is an appropriate statistical method for the comparison of two samples

(2) $p < 0.05$ indicates a 5 percent chance of being wrong

(3) a p value of 0.01 indicates a greater probability that a difference exists than does a value of 0.05

(4) analysis of variance is an appropriate statistical method for comparison of three groups

534. The standard error of the mean (SEM)

(1) is usually a larger number than the standard deviation of the mean

(2) increases with increased size of the sample

(3) should not be confused with standard error, which has a different meaning

(4) is ambiguous unless the sample size is reported

535. True statements include

(1) type I error refers to erroneously concluding that there is a difference when none actually exists

(2) type II error refers to not identifying a difference when one actually exists

(3) the ability of a statistical test to detect a difference is termed *power*

(4) type II error usually occurs with a very large sample size

536. The line isolation monitor (LIM)

(1) protects against microshock hazard

(2) "isolates" an electronically malfunctioning machine by cutting off power to it

(3) typically rings when a brand-new piece of equipment is used for the first time and is the only situation for which the alarm can be ignored

(4) sounds an alarm when ungrounded power becomes grounded

POSITIONING
AND SAFETY

ANSWERS

523. **The answer is C.** (Miller, 4/e. pp 2626–2631.) Electrical power to the OR is an ungrounded, isolated system achieved by an isolation transformer. Therefore, the ground (e.g., the OR floor) is not part of the circuit, as is the case in a grounded system. In this latter system, physical contact with a shorted piece of equipment will complete a circuit (i.e., current from equipment, through person making contact with equipment, to ground). In an isolated system this will not occur, as the ground is not part of the circuit. The LIM functions to continuously monitor this isolation of the electrical power. Equipment with short circuits (e.g., balloon pump) plugged into an isolated system will continue to function, but the LIM will sound an alarm. The "grounding pad" is an unfortunate misnomer used in reference to the Bovie. The patient should never be grounded.

524. **The answer is C.** (Barash, 3/e. p 137. Miller, 4/e. pp 2630–2632.) An understanding of electrical safety in the operating room requires knowledge of Ohm's law, which may be stated several ways. One formulation is electromotive force (V) is equal to the product of current (I) and resistance (R).

525. **The answer is D.** (Miller, 4/e. p 2688.) Universal precautions do not apply to saliva unless it is visibly contaminated by blood. Gloves should be worn, however, when one is working in a patient's mouth. Universal precautions should be applied to all patients regardless of suspicion of infectivity. Blood and body fluids containing visible blood should be considered infectious, as should vaginal, cerebrospinal, synovial, pleural, peritoneal, pericardial, and amniotic fluids. Universal precautions need not be applied to feces, nasal secretions, sputum, sweat, tears, urine, and vomitus unless there is visible blood (although common sense should be used in handling these substances). HIV infection has not been demonstrated to be transmitted via sputum or saliva. Eye shields as well as gloves, gowns, and masks should be used when appropriate.

526. **The answer is D.** (Miller, 4/e. p 761.) Assuming a normal distribution, 95 percent of the data pairs will fall within two standard deviations of the differences.

527. **The answer is B.** (Miller, 4/e. pp 2689–2694.) The addictive potentials of sufentanil and fentanyl are extremely high. There have been anecdotal reports of addiction after a single use of sufentanil. Use of 50 to 100 mL of fentanyl and 10 to 20 mL of sufentanil is not uncommon in an addicted physician. Easy access to drugs is a contributing factor to the high rate of drug addiction among anesthesiologists. However, drug addicts usually can outsmart any drug-tracking system. Qualified board-eligible physicians who are in recovery may take the board examinations, although certification may be delayed and is considered on an individual basis.

528. **The answer is A (1, 2, 3).** (Miller, 4/e. pp 577–578.) Choices 1 and 2 are true for reasons identical to those which apply to the normal upright or supine lung. An anesthetized patient has a perfusion gradient similar to that of an awake patient, but the ventilation inequality between the two lungs is much more pronounced than in an awake patient regardless of whether ventilation is spontaneous or controlled. This ventilation inequality is due to loss of functional residual capacity (FRC) in an anesthetized patient, which causes diminished alveolar compliance in the dependent lung so that relatively more of the tidal volume goes to the nondependent (and poorly perfused) lung. An anesthetized patient has relatively less ventilation to the dependent lung owing to its reduced compliance, its lack of assistance from an actively contracting diaphragm, and its difficulty in expansion caused by the weight of the mediastinum resting above it and the abdomen pushing upon it.

529. **The answer is D (4).** (Miller, 4/e. pp 1057–1060, 1071.) Ulnar nerve injuries are the most common and usually are due to improper padding at the elbow. The common peroneal nerve is the nerve likely to be injured by stirrups; inability to dorsiflex the foot (footdrop) results. Arms should be abducted no more than 90°. Many anesthetics depress compensatory autonomic responses (such as vasoconstriction) to position changes. This results in pooling of blood in gravity-dependent areas with reductions in venous return to the heart and hypotension.

530. **The answer is D (4).** (Miller, 4/e. pp 1063, 1072, 2054.) The area of sensory loss in choice 1 best describes an injury to the lateral femoral cutaneous nerve, which can result from compression by stirrups but not by forceps. Hands should be supinated to avoid ulnar nerve injury. Alopecia can occur after long operations, but the etiology is pressure on the scalp. The head should be turned from time to time to avoid prolonged pressure in one spot. Zone 3 of the lung, where perfusion is greatest, shifts cephalad to poorly ventilated areas in the Trendelenburg position. Furthermore, abdominal contents move cephalad, which compresses alveoli at the bases of the lungs. Both factors produce ventilation-perfusion inequality.

531. **The answer is D (4).** (Miller, 4/e. pp 1367, 1373.) Unanesthetized subjects experience vasoconstriction when body temperature decreases by about 0.4°C. In anesthetized subjects, vasoconstriction does not occur until body temperature decreases by 2.5°C. While beneficial against brain ischemia, mild hypothermia adversely affects wound healing and platelet function. Hypothermia immediately after induction of general anesthesia is due to redistribution of heat within the body and is difficult to prevent.

532. **The answer is C (2, 4).** (Gregory, 2/e. p 496. Miller, 4/e. pp 463, 1376, 1371. Kaplan, 2/e. p 421.) Arrhythmias often occur as temperatures reach and fall below 30 to 32°C. They can be ventricular or atrial, rapid or slow. Osborne waves are "J" point elevations seen with hypothermia. Hypothermia in newborns is associated with hypoventilation and acidosis. A left-shielded oxyhemoglobin dissociation curve produces relative tissue hypoxia.

533. **The answer is E (all).** (Miller, 4/e. pp 763–767.) All these descriptions are accurate.

534. **The answer is D (4).** (Miller, 4/e. pp 761–762.) SEM is standard deviation divided by the square root of the sample size. It is usually numerically smaller than SD. It is often referred to as standard error. SEM can mistakenly be interpreted as small variability of the population studied if it is reported without disclosure of sample size.

535. **The answer is A (1, 2, 3).** (Miller, 4/e. p 763.) Type II error usually occurs with small sample sizes. With small sample sizes, a real difference between groups may not be detectable.

536. **The answer is D (4).** (Miller, 4/e. p 2626.) The line isolation monitor offers no protection against microshock; its threshold for current leakage is 2 mA, while microshock occurs at currents well below that. The line isolation monitor simply monitors whether an ungrounded power system remains so. If it becomes grounded, the LIM will sound an alarm but will not discontinue power. When a new piece of equipment activates the LIM alarm, it should be immediately disconnected and checked.

RECOVERY

Directions: Each question below contains five suggested responses. Select the **one best** response to each question.

537. The most common cause of hypoxemia in the postanesthesia care unit (PACU) is

(A) narcotic overdose
(B) hypoventilation
(C) a low cardiac output state
(D) increased intrapulmonary right-to-left shunting
(E) increased metabolic oxygen consumption

538. Initial management of an agitated patient in the PACU includes all the following EXCEPT

(A) assessment for gastric distention
(B) assessment of oxygenation and ventilation
(C) assessment of a full bladder
(D) treatment with a short-acting benzodiazepine
(E) relief of pain and patient reassurance

539. Etiologic factors that contribute to nausea and vomiting in the PACU include all the following EXCEPT

(A) type of surgical procedure
(B) anesthetic technique
(C) nitrous oxide
(D) postoperative pain
(E) gastric distention

540. The risk of postoperative renal failure is increased in all the following settings EXCEPT

(A) surgical procedure on the heart or great vessels
(B) trauma surgery
(C) major biliary surgery
(D) posterior fossa craniotomies
(E) sepsis

Directions: Each question below contains four suggested responses of which **one or more** is correct. Select

(A)	if	**1, 2, and 3**	are correct
(B)	if	**1 and 3**	are correct
(C)	if	**2 and 4**	are correct
(D)	if	**4**	is correct
(E)	if	**1, 2, 3, and 4**	are correct

541. Primary maneuvers in the treatment of airway obstruction in the PACU include

(1) supplemental oxygen administration
(2) backward head tilt and anterior displacement of the mandible
(3) insertion of a nasal airway
(4) mask ventilation and administration of 20 mg succinylcholine IV

542. Postoperative nausea and vomiting can be controlled by

(1) droperidol 75 μg/kg
(2) ondansetron 4 mg
(3) metoclopramide
(4) scopolamine patches in the PACU

543. Causes of postoperative unconsciousness include

(1) profound neuromuscular blockade
(2) abnormalities in electrolytes
(3) deep hypothermia
(4) thrombotic CVAs

544. Severe hypothermia in a patient who presents for admission to the PACU has been implicated in

(1) new onset of seizure activity
(2) myocardial dysfunction and dysrhythmias
(3) acute renal failure
(4) bleeding diathesis

545. Common causes of postoperative hemorrhage include

(1) coagulation factory deficiency
(2) thrombocytopenia
(3) primary fibrinolysis
(4) loss of vascular integrity (surgical bleeding)

546. Discharge criteria for outpatient surgery include

(1) no bleeding or oozing from the wound site
(2) return of sympathetic nervous function after spinal or epidural anesthesia
(3) ability to void after urologic procedure
(4) duration of surgery less than 3 h

547. The differential diagnosis of a patient in the recovery room who is stridorous 1.5 h after subtotal thyroidectomy (and has not received any medications in the recovery room) should include

(1) infection of the surgical wound, which is causing neck edema and tracheal compression
(2) bilateral recurrent laryngeal nerve (RLN) damage
(3) acute hypercalcemia, which is causing laryngospasm
(4) opioid or muscle relaxant overdose

548. True statements about hypotensive shock include

(1) cardiogenic shock is characterized by increased pulmonary artery occlusion pressure (PAOP) and a low cardiac index

(2) septic shock may present with sudden, irreversible ventricular dysrhythmias

(3) hypovolemic shock manifests as low PAOP with a normal cardiac index

(4) septic shock has low PAOP and cardiac output with high systemic vascular resistance

549. Trimethaphan for treatment of postoperative hypertension can lead to

(1) ganglionic blockade, preventing reflex tachycardia

(2) tachyphylaxis after 12 h of use

(3) ileus and urinary retention

(4) reflex increase in pulse pressure

550. Physiologic adverse effects of postoperative pain include

(1) increased skeletal muscle spasm

(2) stimulation of sympathetic neural pathways

(3) hypothalamic stimulation

(4) hypermotility of the GI and urinary tracts

551. True statements concerning postanesthetic tremor during recovery from anesthesia include

(1) postoperative tremors have both tonic and clonic components

(2) postoperative tremors most commonly occur at end-tidal isoflurane concentrations less than 0.1%

(3) postoperative tremors can be treated effectively by warming the skin surface

(4) all opioids at doses equipotent to 10 to 30 mg meperidine can effectively treat postoperative tremors

552. Preemptive pain treatment may

(1) control perception of postoperative pain

(2) decrease functional changes in the CNS, leading to more acute pain

(3) give prophylaxis against chronic pain states

(4) eliminate phantom limb pain in amputees

RECOVERY

---

537. The answer is D. (Miller, 4/e. p 2312.) The most common cause of hypoxemia in the PACU is an increase in intrapulmonary right-to-left shunting. This most commonly results from atelectasis. The differential diagnosis includes bronchial obstruction caused by secretions or blood, an unknown endobronchial intubation, pneumothorax, cardiogenic or noncardiogenic pulmonary edema, the surgical procedure (upper abdominal or thoracic), and situations in which the closing capacity is greater than the functional residual capacity (obesity or old age). Hypoxia caused by right-to-left shunting may be due to a single cause but most often is due to a combination of these factors.

538. The answer is D. (Miller, 4/e. p 2320.) Hypoxemia and hypercarbia are a common cause of agitation. Administration of a benzodiazepine in an agitated postoperative patient before adequate diagnosis is very dangerous. Benzodiazepines may cause increased respiratory depression and worsen agitation. In patients who are agitated secondary to pain, administration of a benzodiazepine will exacerbate the agitation.

539. The answer is C. (Miller, 4/e. p 2321.) Nitrous oxide has not been implicated in increased incidence of nausea and vomiting postoperatively. The most important factor causing nausea and vomiting is the type of surgery performed rather than the anesthetic technique. Laparoscopic procedures and strabismus surgery lead to the highest incidence of postoperative nausea and vomiting. Other causes include pain, a full bladder, gastric distention, and a vasovagal incident when ambulating. Nausea and vomiting are very uncomfortable and lead to prolonged stays in the PACU. Any one of a number of antiemetics may limit postoperative nausea and vomiting.

540. The answer is D. (Rogers, pp 2371, 2225, 306.) Acute oliguric failure in a postoperative patient has a mortality of 50 percent. The etiology is broken down broadly into prerenal, renal, and postrenal causes. Aside from the settings mentioned, groups at risk include patients who have received massive transfusion therapy, elderly patients, and patients who already have underlying renal disease. Posterior fossa craniotomies have not been implicated as an independent risk factor for postoperative acute renal failure.

541. **The answer is A (1, 2, 3).** (Miller, 4/e. p 231.) The most common cause of airway obstruction in the PACU is the tongue's sagging in the oropharynx. If there is still airway obstruction despite all the corrective maneuvers described, laryngospasm must be considered. With laryngospasm, one will often hear a characteristic crowing sound emitted from the upper airway when ventilation is attempted. Treatment consists of positive pressure ventilation by mask. If the laryngospasm is not relieved, 20 mg succinylcholine IV should be given while supporting ventilation. Other rare causes of upper airway obstruction include foreign bodies (such as teeth), postextubation croup, and vocal cord paresis.

542. **The answer is A (1, 2, 3).** (Miller, 4/e. pp 2321–2322.) Each of the first three drugs can aid in prophylaxis against nausea and vomiting as well as be effective after nausea has occurred. Scopolamine patches must be placed several hours ahead of time to be effective.

543. **The answer is E (all).** (Miller, 4/e. pp 2319–2320.) In addition, hypoglycemia, intraoperative hypoxemia, raised ICP, and residual anesthetic effects can lead to decreased consciousness postoperatively.

544. **The answer is C (2, 4).** (Miller, 4/e. pp 1371, 1376.) Hypothermia has not been implicated in the new onset of seizure activity or directly in acute renal failure. It does cause shivering, which may increase oxygen consumption by as much as five times the norm. This in turn requires an increase in cardiac output, which may lead to dysrhythmias and myocardial dysfunction. Platelet function may be impaired in severe hypothermia and lead to a bleeding diathesis.

545. **The answer is D (4).** (Miller, 4/e. pp 1626–1628.) Clotting factor deficiencies are rare causes of postoperative hemorrhage. Low percentages of clotting factors on the order of 20 to 30 percent are needed for normal coagulation. Primary fibrinolysis and thrombocytopenia are also rare causes of postoperative hemorrhage; the latter may be caused most frequently by massive dilution from severe bleeding or massive consumption, as occurs with disseminated intravascular coagulation (DIC). The major cause of postoperative hemorrhage is loss of vascular integrity, i.e., surgical bleeding or poor hemostasis.

546. **The answer is A (1, 2, 3).** (Miller, 4/e. pp 2239–2240.) Duration of surgery is not a consideration for discharge after outpatient surgery as long as the other listed criteria are met. In addition, there are other discharge criteria, which include stable vital signs, no worsening or new occurrence of symptoms related to the particular surgery, ability to tolerate fluid with minimal nausea, intact neurovascular function after extremity surgery, normal neurologic status, ability to ambulate with minimal dizziness, and easily controlled postoperative pain.

547. **The answer is C (2, 4).** (Rogers, pp 2039, 2042.) Wound infection would not occur this early. However, hemorrhage with neck swelling should be considered, and the neck should be inspected. Sutures should be opened immediately if the airway is compromised by an expanding hematoma. It is more probable that unilateral RLN damage would occur, which usually causes hoarseness, not stridor, but bilateral involvement is a possibility. Inadvertent removal of parathyroids can cause acute hypocalcemia with generalized muscle spasm, including laryngospasm. This usually does not occur until 24 to 72 h postoperatively. At 1.5 h after surgery, opioid or muscle relaxant overdose is unlikely. However, if the patient received naloxone at the end of surgery during which a long-acting opioid was employed, rebound opioid effect can occur at about this time. Similarly, if a deep neuromuscular blockade with a long-acting muscle relaxant was used, a rebound relaxant effect could occur at about this time as the neostigmine wears off, especially in the presence of hypoventilation (with a concomitant respiratory acidosis), as this will augment neuromuscular blockade.

548. **The answer is A (1, 2, 3).** (Miller, 4/e. pp 2216–2218.)

	PAOP	CI	SVR
Hypovolemic	↓	↓	↑
Cardiogenic	↑	↓	↑
Septic	↑	↑	↓

Treatment should focus on the cause of the hypotension. Hypovolemia requires volume. Cardiogenic shock requires optimization of preload as well as inotropic support. Septic shock requires pressor support, crystalloid volume, and treatment of the sepsis. Prolonged low diastolic pressure may lead to myocardial ischemia and ventricular dysrhythmias. PA monitoring is an invaluable diagnostic tool in these situations.

549. **The answer is A (1, 2, 3).** (Miller, 4/e. p 2319.) Ganglionic blockade by trimethaphan prevents the reflex tachycardia seen with nitroprusside but can cause ileus and urinary retention. Tachyphylaxis is common after 12 to 24 h of infusion. However, there is no reflex increase in pulse pressure as can be seen with nitroprusside.

550. **The answer is A (1, 2, 3).** (Miller, 4/e. pp 2327–2328.) Increases in skeletal muscle tone and spasm can lead to increased O_2 consumption and lactate production. Similarly, sympathetic and hypothalamic stimulation lead to tachycardia, increased heart work, and increased O_2 consumption. Pain usually causes hypomotility of the GI and urinary tracts, leading to ileus and urinary retention.

551. **The answer is B (1, 3).** (Miller, 4/e. pp 1372, 2322.) Postoperative tremor most commonly occurs at end-tidal isoflurane concentrations of 0.1 to 0.2%. Meperidine is the only opioid that has been found to be efficacious in the treatment of postoperative tremors.

552. **The answer is E (all).** (Miller, 4/e. p 2329.) It is thought that rather than solely treating pain after it occurs, prevention of its occurrence can lead to a decrease in the overall sensation of pain. Nerve blocks or epidural opioids before surgery can interrupt the noxious stimuli sensed by the CNS. This may prevent the sensitization of the CNS to pain, which can cause postoperative pain to be perceived as even worse than it actually is.

BIBLIOGRAPHY

American Heart Association: *Textbook of Advanced Cardiac Life Support.* American Heart Association, 1994.

Barash PG, Cullen BF, Stoelting RK (eds): *Clinical Anesthesia,* 3/e. Philadelphia, JB Lippincott, 1997.

Cousins MJ, Bridenbaugh PO (eds): *Neural Blockade in Clinical Anesthesia and Management of Pain,* 2/e. Philadelphia, JB Lippincott, 1988.

Firestone LL (ed): *Clinical Anesthesia Procedures of the Massachusetts General Hospital,* 3/e. Boston, Little, Brown, 1988.

Gregory, GA: *Pediatric Anesthesia,* 2/e. Churchill Livingstone, New York, 1989.

Kaplan JA (ed): *Cardiac Anesthesia,* 2/e. Philadelphia, WB Saunders, 1987.

Katz J, Benumof JL: *Anesthesia and Uncommon Diseases,* 3/e. Philadelphia, WB Saunders, 1990.

Miller RD (ed): *Anesthesia,* 4/e. New York, Churchill Livingstone, 1994.

Rogers MC: *Principles and Practice of Anesthesiology.* Mosby Year Book, 1992.

Shnider SM, Levinson G (eds): *Anesthesia for Obstetrics,* 3/e. Baltimore, Williams & Wilkins, 1987.

Stoelting RK: *Pharmacology and Physiology in Anesthetic Practice,* 2/e. Philadelphia, JB Lippincott, 1991.

Stoelting RK, Dierdorf SF, McCammon RL: *Anesthesia and Co-Existing Disease,* 3/e. New York, Churchill Livingstone, 1993.

Wedel DJ: (ed): *Orthopedic Anesthesia,* Churchill Livingstone, 1993.

NOTES

NOTES

NOTES

NOTES

NOTES

ISBN 0-07-015102-4

90000